The Logic of Care

What is good care? In this innovative and compelling book, Annemarie Mol argues that good care has little to do with 'patient choice' and, therefore, creating more opportunities for patient choice will not improve health care.

Although it is possible to treat people who seek professional help as customers or citizens, Mol argues that this undermines ways of thinking and acting crucial to health care. Illustrating the discussion with examples from diabetes clinics and diabetes self care, the book presents the 'logic of care' in a step by step contrast with the 'logic of choice'. She concludes that good care is not a matter of making well-argued individual choices but is something that grows out of collaborative and continuing attempts to attune knowledge and technologies to diseased bodies and complex lives.

Mol does not criticise the practices she encountered in her field work as messy or ad hoc, but makes explicit what it is that motivates them: an intriguing combination of adaptability and perseverance. *The Logic of Care: Health and the problem of patient choice* is crucial reading for all those interested in the theory and practice of care, including sociologists, anthropologists and health-care professionals. It will also speak to policymakers and become a valuable source of inspiration for patient activists.

Annemarie Mol is Socrates Professor of Political Philosophy at the University of Twente, the Netherlands.

The Logic of Care

Health and the problem of patient choice

Annemarie Mol

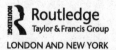

Routledge
Taylor & Francis Group

LONDON AND NEW YORK

First published in 2006 with the title *De logica van het zorgen. Actieve patiënten en de grenzen van het kiezen* by Van Gennep, Amsterdam

Published 2008
by Routledge
2 Park Square, Milton Park, Abingdon, Oxon OX14 4RN

Simultaneously published in the USA and Canada
by Routledge
711 Third Avenue, New York, NY 10017

Routledge is an imprint of the Taylor & Francis Group, an informa business

Translation and adaptation from the Dutch: Peek Language Services and the author.

Changes have also been introduced: there are differences throughout between the English and the Dutch version of this book.

Typeset in Perpetua by Wearset Ltd, Boldon, Tyne and Wear

British Library Cataloguing in Publication Data
A catalogue record for this book is available from the British Library

Library of Congress Cataloging in Publication Data
Mol, Annemarie.
[Logica van het zorgen. English]
The logic of care: health and the problem of patient choice / Annemarie Mol.
p.cm.
Includes bibliographical references.
1. Medical care–Evaluation. 2. Medical care–Quality control. 3. Patient satisfaction. 4. Patients–Civil rights. 5. Diabetes–Treatment–Netherlands–Case studies. I. Title.
[DNLM: 1. Quality of Health Care. 2. Choice Behavior. 3. Diabetes Mellitus–therapy. 4. Patient Care. 5. Personal Autonomy. 6. Professional-Patient Relations. W 84.1 M717L 2008a]
RA399.A1M6513 2008
362.1–dc22   2007047374

ISBN10: 0-415-45342-9 (hbk)
ISBN10: 0-415-45343-7 (pbk)
ISBN10: 0-203-92707-9 (ebk)

ISBN13: 978-0-415-45342-4 (hbk)
ISBN13: 978-0-415-45343-1 (pbk)
ISBN13: 978-0-203-92707-6 (ebk)

For Elisabeth and Johannes

Contents

The hidden brave 82

6 The good in practice   84
    Morality in action 85
    Active patients 91
    Improving health care 96
    Translations 103

    Acknowledgements   109
    Notes   113
    Literature   131
    Index   140

Prologue

In this book I will contrast two ways of dealing with disease. One of these, the logic of care, is the central topic of this book, while the other, the logic of choice, forms its point of contrast. But let me begin by telling some stories. These could be presented either as personal experiences or as ethnographic observations, the difference is not really relevant. Together they index the events that led me to write this book, and they provide a first sense of the concerns that lie behind it.

Story one. It is the early 1980s. On Dutch television a discussion on in vitro fertilisation is about to be broadcast. As a young feminist scholar, studying biomedicine and its techniques, I sit down to watch how the promises and problems of IVF will be staged. No doubt there will be talk about much loved babies. But what about the impressive quantities of hormones that are injected into women in the course of this intervention? Will anyone mention the way that these women's lives are ordered around ovulation and egg-harvesting for months on end? Will the discussion dwell on the fact that parental hope for a child 'of their own' is being fuelled, even though in most cases it is never met? I realise that it is unlikely that any of the guests will contrast the emotional and financial investment made in any Western child with the fact that children in the rest of the world die in large numbers of hunger and infectious diseases. Nor will anyone ask why organising good daycare facilities seems so much less urgent than making babies. Yet I am curious.

After some preliminaries and explanations, the gynaecologist is asked to speak. However, he almost immediately shifts this task to 'the patient'. *His* patient. There she is: a woman who will appeal to many – she could be a professional herself, a feminist even, but also someone who gave up work once she got married. Presenting herself both as suffering and proud, she tells the audience that, yes, indeed, she has so far failed to get pregnant in the usual way. She wants a child very badly. Therefore, whatever the possible risks or drawbacks she is undergoing IVF. It is, she says, her own choice. At this point the camera shifts back to the gynaecologist. Who would be so paternalistic, he says, as to deny this woman her choice? End of discussion. As if it were a magic wand, the term 'choice' has ended the discussion. All the possible advantages and disadvantages of the treatment, all its goods and bads, have been turned into private concerns. They are not to be questioned. Interestingly, the gynaecologist's words come straight out of the abortion debate that had taken place in the Netherlands barely a decade earlier. There it is, the term 'paternalistic', which evokes male arrogance; 'her own' that makes the woman sound courageous; and finally there is 'choice', the very act that turns a person into a subject. What to say? The question of how to counter the magic of the term 'choice' has haunted me ever since.

Story two. Ten years on. I've kept on researching and writing. Now, as a supposedly neutral third party, I am invited to chair a discussion about *choice* and *patient autonomy* between ethicists and psychiatrists. One of the ethicists begins by presenting a case. Briefly: one morning a patient in an open ward of a psychiatric hospital does not want to get up. Question: are you going to allow him to stay in bed or not? (It is implied that 'you' are in the safe position of the psychiatrist, who may offer others the freedom to choose, or not. Somehow the 'you' of medical ethics is never a patient. But that is in parentheses.) Most of the ethicists in the meeting think the case is easy. A person who stays in bed does not harm anyone else. It is the pivotal liberal principle that people are allowed to make their own choices so long as they do not harm others. Let him be, this man, let him make his own choice. One ethicist sees a problem however. What if the person in question is incapable of functioning as a subject of choice, what if he – he's a patient after all – is insane? A discussion about madness ensues. Is a patient in a psychiatric hospital always 'mad' and incapable of making choices? Or is this only the case if he happens to be psychotic, acutely depressed or otherwise overwhelmed by disease? The question of autonomy gets linked up with that of psychiatric diagnosis. Thus the ethicists seem to silence themselves. For when it comes to diagnosis, the psychiatrists are the experts.

However, the psychiatrists present do not seem too worried about diagnosis. They have other concerns. One of them says that, since life in a hospital ward is communal, people have to adapt to shared rules. In a family, he says, you also have to join in for breakfast. Such routines make for a better daily life. Another psychiatrist stresses that people admitted to a psychiatric hospital often have to *learn* to make choices: this is a part of their treatment. So whether this particular patient is up to being confronted with the negative consequences of making a bad choice (no breakfast, no daytime activities) or should be encouraged to get up as a way of protecting him, depends on the stage of his treatment. Further responses go off in other directions. One of them is striking. The retired Professor of Psychotherapy says: it is all a question of money. He reproaches the ethicist who has presented the case for leaving out the institutional context. A dilemma like this, he says, only arises when there are not enough staff: 'On a ward with enough staff, I'd send a nurse to sit next to the patient's bed and ask *why* he does not want to get up. Maybe his wife is not coming for a visit that afternoon. Maybe he feels awful and fears he will never be released from hospital. Take time for him, let him talk.' Someone who does not want to get up, says the psychotherapist, needs care. Offering him the choice of staying in bed is as much a way of neglecting him as is forcing him to get up.

This is helpful. Yes, there is not only a contrast between 'choice' and 'no choice', but also between these two, united in a *logic of choice*, and an altogether different alternative, that of care, something that contrasts with neglect. Might it be possible, I wonder in the days, the years, that follow, to find ways of articulating a *logic of care*?

Story three. It is still the early 1990s. I am pregnant and 36. A national committee of experts in the Netherlands where I live has looked at the statistics and suggested that pregnant women over 35 should have an amniocentesis and thus the option of abortion should their foetus have Down's Syndrome. Given where I am (I have a healthy child and work that fascinates me and it is difficult enough as it is to juggle between them) I follow the advice. I take a day off and go to the hospital where I also happen to be doing the field work for the book that I am working on at the time. It is slightly strange to shift from the role of observer to that of patient. But I lie down on the examination table and feel the ultrasound probe moving over my belly. Still in my field-work habits, or just to break the silence, I say to the nurse who is preparing the long needle that will be inserted into my womb: 'I hope it all goes okay.' We both know that a small percentage of women have a spontaneous abortion as a result of the procedure. The nurse snaps back: 'Well, it is your own choice.'

Back home I dutifully sit down on the couch, legs up, to reduce the chance of the threatened spontaneous abortion. But I also start to make notes for what turns out to be field work after all, albeit for some future book. I wonder what the nurse might have said that would have fitted a logic of care. 'Let's indeed hope it goes well'; or 'Most of the time there's no problem'; or 'Are you worried about it?' She might have touched me in a kind way. And she might even have used the moment to encourage me to behave and say: 'You may want to have a quiet afternoon, then.' But instead she illustrates beautifully how mobilising the logic of choice can lead to poor care. It can shift the weight of everything that goes wrong onto the shoulders of the patient-chooser.

Over the last twenty years, 'choice' and more particularly 'patient choice' has attracted ever more public attention. Its public appeal has increased too. Over the same period I hit upon more and more reasons for doubting it. Thus, when early in the new century ZON/Mw, the Netherlands Organisation for Health Research and Development, offered grants for studies intended to 'increase the possibilities for patient choice', I wrote an application. It stated that, if it is compared with 'force', then 'choice' is more often than not a great good. But what about comparing it with 'care'? Is 'care' a soft form of 'force' or might something entirely different be going on? I got the grant which made it possible to investigate a specific set of care activities in more detail than provided in the examples above. I analysed them again and again and then gradually wrote this book. It argues that, indeed, in care practices something entirely different is going on. Care has a logic of its own. The logic of care. How to talk about it?

1   Two logics

Individual choice is a widely celebrated ideal. This is hardly strange: who likes to be dominated by others? And yet this book starts out from doubts about this ideal. I do not question choice in general, but rather the generalisation of choice. Other ideals, like 'good care', suffer from this. In health care, on which this book concentrates, 'patient choice' and 'good care' may sometimes complement each other, but more often they clash. Practices designed to foster 'patient choice' erode existing practices that were established to ensure 'good care'. People who are directly involved in health care (as professionals or as patients) have sad stories to tell about this. However attractive it may sound, when it comes to it, 'patient choice' does not always lead to the expected improvements. Why not? Where do things go wrong? To tackle these questions, I will not discuss the merits of the ideals of 'individual choice' and 'good care' in and of themselves, in isolation. Instead I will unravel some exemplary practices with which they are linked.[1]

In scholarly discussions about health care, 'care' is often distinguished from 'cure'. If this is done, the first term, 'care', is used for activities such as washing, feeding or dressing wounds, that are done to make daily life more bearable. The second term, 'cure', resonates with the possibility of healing, and is applied to interventions in the course of a disease. In the present book I deliberately avoid making this distinction. In practice, after all, the activities categorised as 'care' and 'cure' overlap. (Caring) food and (curing) drugs may have similar effects on a body. Caringly dressing a wound may help its cure. What is more, nowadays many of the diseases that send people to their doctors are chronic in character. A so-called cure of such conditions does not lead to recovery but instead makes life more bearable: it is a form of care. Thus, even if the interventions in the lives and bodies of people with chronic diseases are often knowledge-intensive and technology-dependent, there are good reasons for calling them care. Which is what I'll do here – I will skip the term 'cure' and talk only of 'care'. In the process that word will slightly change its meaning.

The practices I have analysed in order to compare 'patient choice' and 'good care' are those of the treatment of, and life with, diabetes in the Netherlands. Thus the stories I tell are highly specific. They are local. That does not mean their significance is local. I will not begin to explore what can be transported from this particular site and situation and what cannot. But my hope is that, not despite, but thanks to, their specificity, these stories are strong enough to get across the importance of 'good care'. This is an important ideal and we had better not throw it out in order to haul in 'individual choice'. A caution. If I talk about 'good care' using 'diabetes care in the Netherlands' as my case, this does not mean that the particular clinic that I investigated, or Dutch health care overall, are wonderful. There is a lot left to improve. But, and this is my point, continuing to empha-sise patient choice will not bring about the improvements hoped for. Introducing patient choice into health care does not (finally) make space for us, its patients. Instead, it alters daily practices in ways that do not necessarily fit well with the intricacies of our diseases. My argument is that the tradition of care contains more suitable reper-toires for handling life with a disease. Instead of frustrating these by dreaming of choice, it would be wiser to try to improve care on its own terms. In its own terms. But in what language to speak of care and its specificities? The ideal of good care is silently incorporated in practices and does not speak for itself. Given that it is under threat, it is time to put it into words. That is what I set out to do here. In this book I talk about the treatment of, and life with, diabetes, while seeking words that allow me to do so. The aim is to articulate the specificities of good care so that we may talk about it.[2]

Clichés of the West

In this book you will find snapshot stories about the treatment of, and life with, diabetes inside and outside the hospital. Thus you will learn how Mrs Jansen is taught to prick her finger in order to get a few drops of blood. She learns to squeeze these drops onto a stick and insert this into a blood sugar monitor in order to determine her blood sugar level. Mr Zomer is also encouraged to do this, but it appears that he cannot incorporate self-measurement into his daily life. Why not? Then there is Lies Henstra, who will explain to her interviewer that she eats too much because she comes from a family of food lovers. You will encounter a diabetes nurse, who wonders which make of blood sugar monitor might fit into each patient's daily life best. And there are doctors, too. In this book they are fused into 'the doctor', who tries to help her patients to creatively adjust useful technologies and daily lives to each other. Mobilising events and quotes, I will gradually flesh out 'good care'. But before I start to do this I would like to invite you on a detour. I want to set the stage. For the stage on which 'choice' and 'care' clash, is not confined to the consulting room and the daily lives of patients. It is far larger. One might as well say it is 'the West'.

Individual choice is not only celebrated as an ideal in health care. It surfaces everywhere. In discussions about organising schools, raising children, finding work, building houses, cooking food, making music, financing the media – the list goes on and on. People should not enjoy their autonomy at the expense of others, but autonomous they should be. And this is not just a strong moral preoccupation. The difference between autonomy and heteronomy has also come to mark the difference between 'the West' and 'the Others'. In this context, 'the West' is typecast as a place/time where people make individual choices, while 'the Others' are said to be embedded in their communities. While God, tradition and the collective give meaning and coherence to 'their' lives, 'we Westerners', by contrast, are supposed to have been free of such restrictive ties since the Enlightenment. The specificities tend to be left in the dark. Did 'our' liberation take place two centuries ago, at the time of Voltaire and his friends; or not until the 1960s, with youth revolt and the pill? And who exactly belongs to the 'we' of 'the West'? Only truly secularised people, or also those who have confined religion to their private lives? Only rationalists, or men, or the well educated, or everyone who lives in a so-called Western country? Do the fundamentalists in the southern states of the US belong? And what about the inhabitants of Singapore, Rio de Janeiro, Johannesburg or Beirut? So long as such questions are not actually asked, the demarcation of the 'we' remains fuzzy and taken for granted. What counts is that 'we' are individualised and autonomous. It is this that makes 'us' modern and belong to 'the West'.

In scholarly literatures, this neo-colonial ideological violence has been met with a variety of critical responses. In various ways, such literatures defend the non-West against the caricatures that circulate about it. Some authors argue that 'self-hood' in the non-Western culture they happen to know about, may not quite be 'individualism', but is nothing like 'immersion in the collective' either.[3] Others talk of the people who worked (and died young) on sugar plantations and long-distance sailing ships, in harbours and emerging factories, in order to provide the material conditions for the individualisation of some – preciously few – of their contemporaries.[4] Yet other authors describe sites and situations where 'individualisation' would not have worked. Take West Africa: while people in the coffee houses of London, the salons of Paris and the stock markets of Amsterdam, celebrated personal liberty, people in West Africa had to rely on each other for protection against (English, French, Dutch) slave traders. A solitary individual would have had nowhere to hide.[5] In ways like this post-colonial studies have criticised self-satisfied Enlightenment fantasies. Here I would like to contribute to that line of work. However, I will not do so by countering more bad clichés about 'the Others', but by readjusting bad clichés about 'the West'.[6]

Are 'we', in 'the West', indeed autonomous individuals? The answer is: no, 'we' are not. This is hardly an original statement: it has been argued many times. Sociologists have emphasised that all humans are born naked and helpless and depend on others for their survival for years. Even as adults Westerners are interdependent – all the more since they no longer cultivate their own food, sew their own clothes, or bury their own dead. Some sociologists have studied how in actual practice people in 'free societies' make their choices. They have found that making choices takes a lot of energy, energy that not everybody has to spare or likes to spend on it. They have also found that 'we' end up choosing remarkably similar things. Indeed, some scholars have argued that autonomy is not the opposite of heteronomy at all. Instead, they say, making people long for choices and invest a lot in making them, is a disciplining technique.[7]

So 'we' in 'the West' may not have as much 'choice' as we think, or not like it as much, or not use it in such a way that we end up

doing other things than other people, or we may not be freed by
having choices to make, but tricked. What is more, besides the ideal
of 'choice', there are many others circulating in 'the West': for
instance solidarity, justice, mutual respect and care. There it is, care.
The present book is obviously by no means the first to stress the
importance of care. This has been done before, in many different
ways. Theologians have cast care as a selfless activity, inspired by
charity and love. Anthropologists have contrasted the fluid circulation of care with the metrically calculated reciprocity implied in
exchange. They have cast care as a gift. Within the sociology of
work, the care and devotion with which many people throw themselves into their work has been shown to fit badly with the formality
of employment contracts. And then there is the care of parents for
their children. How is this different from and how does it combine
with paid work? Or, another question, is only (maternal) warmth
appropriate to care or is (paternal) discipline equally essential?
Finally, care is discussed within ethics. Care ethicists claim that 'good
care' is not an ideal that can be defended in general terms, as a
matter of principle (in the way that the ethical tradition has sought to
defend an ideal like justice). Instead it is something that people
shape, invent and adapt, time and again, in everyday practices.[8]

Each of these short sentences points to a bookcase. Jointly, the theological, anthropological, sociological, pedagogical and ethical versions
of care underscore the fact that 'the West' is not simply Enlightened.
It does not just celebrate rationality, autonomy and choice, but has a
rich and multi-layered care tradition as well. I need not argue this, it
has been done already. And yet there is something I would like to add.
By unravelling the specificities of care in the case of daily life with diabetes, it is possible to disentangle 'care' from an all too immediate
association with kindness, dedication and generosity. The point is not
that kindness, dedication and generosity are irrelevant to daily life.
They are crucial.[9] But as long as care is primarily associated with
'tender love', it may be cast as something that is opposed to technology. A pre-modern remainder in a modern world. Maybe such care
can be added as a friendly extra, maybe it gets eaten up by technology,
but in either case the two are mutually exclusive. But is this true, is
care *other* to technology? Is the first humane and friendly, while the
second is strategic and depends on rationality alone? This is precisely
where I want to interfere. The care that I will come to talk about, is

not opposed to, but includes, technology. And the technology that I will come to talk about is not transparent and predictable, but has to be handled with care.[10]

'The West' (wherever it may begin or end) has never been homogeneous. Alongside its many horrors, it contains an amalgam of ideals, that of 'good care' among them. To deny this is a form of internal colonisation. It simplifies 'the West' and reduces it to only one of its traditions – which, by declaring it to be dominant, is made to be so ever more. This frustrates good care, contributes to the marginalisation of patients, and makes it difficult to think about, let alone attend to, the body and its diseases. It also helps to hide neglect – a word that risks disappearing from our vocabulary. Finally, it contributes to widening the gap between 'the West' and 'the Others', where instead we would do better to face the problems we share (such as viruses that run wild, or the ecological limits of our life on earth) – or to explore other contrasts (such as those between rich and poor; or between healthy people and people who have intestinal infections or malaria, are hungry, or bound to die from AIDS). This then is both the global context of, and a major drive behind, this book. I like the good food that I eat and my warm, safe bed. But I do not want to be part of a 'West' that alienates me from 'the Others' by making me afraid of being bossed around while, at the same time, failing to address neglect. Articulating what 'good care' entails is an attempt to escape from that unwelcome embrace. It seeks to counter the internal colonisation of all kinds of Western traditions by the single ideal of choice and the rationalism that it is tied up with. Thus, while I will tell you stories that are local and specific, they are set on a large stage. They start out from daily life with diabetes in the Netherlands, but they seek to interfere not only with health care, but also with emptied out versions of technology, all too beautiful dreams about Reason, and one-dimensional clichés about 'the West'.

Active patients

That the ideal of individual choice is so enthusiastically drawn into health care is not only due to its current general popularity in 'the West'. It also has to do with the specificities of health care. If patients visit a doctor, or so the story goes, they are all too often observed,

touched and tested, without having the chance to speak for themselves. As patients we are treated as objects and made passive. This is
a bad practice that should be stopped. Patients deserve to be heard.
They should be respected as subjects who have the right to make the
crucial choices about their own lives for themselves. This is a serious
argument. If I venture to raise doubts about the ideal of patient
choice then I have to respond to it. And so I will. Here, as a first step
in providing that response, I want to distinguish my own doubts
about choice from two other, more common concerns.

The more widespread of these has it that choice may be a great
ideal, but only in situations in which people are indeed able to make
their own choices. When they are patients, people often lack this
ability. If you are brought into the emergency ward in a coma you are
far from autonomous. If you have a high temperature, you ramble. If
you have just found out that you have an aggressive form of cancer,
you are likely to be frightened and confused and may well want
someone else to make decisions for you. In reaction to such examples,
proponents of the ideal of patient choice insist that not all diseases
(disabilities, difficulties) are so overwhelming. Someone in a wheelchair may be unable to walk, but is as able to make choices as the next
person. People with diabetes are no less decisive than people whose
bodies produce their own insulin – so long as their blood sugar levels
are normal. And even if you have just heard that you have cancer, you
may well regain your ability to choose fairly quickly if your doctors
take the necessary time and effort to talk calmly with you. That there
are exceptional situations in which patients are temporarily unable to
decide is no reason to deny the ability to choose to everyone who is a
patient.[11]

A second widespread way of doubting the ideal of choice is to
point out that when it comes to it almost nobody (ill or healthy) is
any good at it. It is difficult for all of us to weigh up the advantages
and disadvantages of one uncertain future against another. We tend
to make incorrect assessments, for instance: to almost everyone a 20
per cent chance of success sounds a lot better than an 80 per cent
chance of failure. We also use fear as our advisor, or let other emotions cloud our judgements. Added to this, many of us lack the
material resources required to choose. The choice of going for a
swim every morning means little if you never learned to swim; if the
swimming pool is too far away or costs too much; or if you have

small children or sick family members to look after. Here, again, proponents of choice have an answer. They stress that the conditions under which 'choice' makes sense should indeed be given more attention. They say that the fact that the conditions enabling people to make informed choices are often not met is no reason to dismiss the ideal.[12]

In both of these discussions the central question is whether people are able to make choices or not. Maybe healthy people are, while people with a disease are not; or maybe some people with a disease are, but not all of them; or maybe everyone can choose if only the relevant conditions are met; and then again, it might be that, when it comes to it, nobody is able to choose. In this book I will avoid this issue. Instead of focusing on the abilities of people, I will talk about the practices in which people are involved. Instead of asking who should make given choices, I will take a step back and consider 'situations of choice'. For these are not self-evidently given. In what kinds of practices do 'situations of choice' arise? By shifting focus in this way it becomes possible to show that the ideal of choice carries a whole world with it: a specific mode of organising action and inter-action; of understanding bodies, people and daily lives; of dealing with knowledge and technologies; of distinguishing between good and bad; and so on. Instead of hinging on people's limited abilities, my doubt has to do with that entire world. A world infused with what I will call the *logic of choice*. It does not offer a superior way of living. More specifically: it does not offer a way of living superior to the life that may be led in a world infused by the alternative that this book seeks to articulate: the *logic of care*.

In response to the argument that choice, finally, liberates patients from the passivity into which they were forced, this book seeks to show that in care practices patients are not passive at all. They are active. However, they do not primarily figure as subjects of choice, but as the subjects of all kinds of activities. The logic of care is not preoccupied with our will, and with what we may opt for, but con-centrates on what we do. Patients tend to do a lot. The people with diabetes whom you will encounter in this book inject their own insulin, measure their own blood sugar levels, count the carbohy-drates they eat, calibrate their exercise and take care of themselves in many other ways as well. This is not to say that engaging in such activities is attractive. It may well be tedious. The crucial question therefore, is not how active we are, but what kinds of activities we engage in. Treatment practices tend to be demanding. What exactly do they demand? What do active patients have to do and what must they abstain from? If we want to improve health care, these are the questions we need to address. Instead of either pushing professionals back into their cage, or allowing them to do whatever they like, it is better to open up and share the crucial substantive questions publicly. How to live well, what to die from, and how, thus, to shape good care?[13]

The method

In my attempts to articulate the logic of care I drew on a variety of resources. I took the term 'logic' from philosophy and ran away with it.[14] There is a risk in using a word like 'logic' when talking of practices. It might seem to suggest that those practices are so coherent that everything within them is firmly defined by everything else. Let me insist that this is not the case. Unexpected things always happen. A lot of creativity is involved in any practice. And yet: locally, some things are more comprehensible than others. Events somehow tend to fit together, there are affinities between them. This is what the term 'logic' is meant to evoke. In this sense it resembles the French 'discours', which is usually translated as 'discourse' in English. In a discourse, words, materialities and practices hang together in a specific, historically and culturally situated way. Another term, 'modes of ordering', resonates in the background as well. 'Modes of ordering' make discourses multiple and mobile. 'Modes' is a plural: it invites a comparison of different ways of thinking and acting that co-exist in a single time and place. 'Ordering', derived from the verb rather than the noun, calls up a process: it suggests that the activity of ordering involves a continuous effort, and that it may always fail.[15]

However, I do not talk about 'discourses' or 'modes of ordering' here, but deliberately use the term 'logic'. This is because my concern is not with the ways in which socio-material orderings come into being and establish themselves, nor with the power involved in that process. Instead, I am after the rationality, or rather the rationale, of the practices I am studying. Here the term 'logic' helps. It asks for something that one might also call a style. It invites the exploration of what it is appropriate or logical to do in some site or situation, and what is not. It seeks a local, fragile and yet pertinent coherence. This coherence is not necessarily obvious to the people involved. It need not even be verbally available to them. It may be implicit: embedded in practices, buildings, habits and machines. And yet, if we want to talk about it, we need to translate a logic into language. This, then, is what I am after. I will make words for, and out of, practices. And I will do so comparatively, using contrast as a way of gaining insight. This book articulates the logic of care through a detailed comparison with the logic of choice.

If logics are embedded in practices, articulating them demands that we go out into the world and immerse ourselves in those practices. This is why, in addition to drawing on philosophy, I have also borrowed from the social sciences: I have done field work. Traditionally, philosophers blocked themselves off from mundanities and tried to argue by reasoning alone. Rational inference was supposed to generate universally valid arguments. And yet the empirical world was included in philosophical texts: in their questions, their quests and their metaphors.[16] And also, of course, in their examples. These might come from just about anywhere: the philosopher's own experiences; discussions with others; the social science literature; novels; movies; newspapers; and so on. The caricature of the genre is the philosopher who tries to get his abstractions across by telling stories about his pipe, his desk and his cat. In ways much like this: 'All living creatures need care. If I did not take care of my cat, did not feed her, she would die.' But maybe the neglected cat in question would simply run away: the experiment was never put into practice.[17] Examples were strictly pedagogical, they were there to help the philosopher explain an argument that had been thought through before the example was brought in to illustrate it.

Philosophers who leave their studies are likely to be surprised. Examining a practice is not a matter of collecting suitable examples, but of learning new lessons. Good case studies inspire theory, shape ideas and shift conceptions. They do not lead to conclusions that are universally valid, but neither do they claim to do so. Instead, the lessons learned are quite specific. If one immerses oneself long enough in a case, one may get a sense of what is acceptable, desirable or called for in a particular setting. This does not mean that it is possible to predict what happens elsewhere or in new situations. Dealing with whatever is different always requires work and logics do not do work. They are not actors, but patterns. Thus, the logic of care articulated here only fits the case that I studied. It does not apply everywhere. This is not to say that its relevance is local. A case study is of wider interest as becomes a part of a trajectory. It offers points of contrast, comparison or reference for other sites and situations. It does not tell us what to expect – or do – anywhere else, but it does suggest pertinent questions. Case studies increase our sensitivity. It is the very specificity of a meticulously studied case that allows us to unravel what remains the same and what changes from one situation to the next.

In order to articulate the logic of care while comparing it with the logic of choice, I have thus examined a case. It is: a variant of the treatment of, and life with, diabetes. To study this case, I have done field work in ethnographic mode. Thus, I have attended consultations of physicians and diabetes nurses in the diabetes outpatient clinic of a university hospital in a medium-sized Dutch town; analysed texts on diabetes from a variety of books, journals and websites aimed at professionals and/or patients; interviewed professionals and patients; and received help from others who also conducted interviews and transcribed them for me.[18] In our interviews we did not ask people about their opinions, but about the events and activities that they were involved in. In this way, the interviews extended ethnographic observation. The interviewees told us about situations where as researchers we had no time or licence to go. Thus, instead of turning professionals and patients into our objects of study, we rather drew upon their skills as co-researchers. They offered us knowledge: knowledge about the treatment of, and life with, diabetes.[19]

All this work generated a lot of material. An anthropologist or a sociologist might have used that material to present reality (or a part of it) as accurately or as grippingly as possible. However, my aim here is different. I do not seek to sketch a faithful image of the events that I or my informants witnessed. Neither do I want to talk about the meanings of these events for those involved in them. Instead of following the interpretations of my informants, I want to add an interpretation of my own. Instead of relating the perspectives of others, I seek to offer a new perspective. Thus I have worked with my materials in the way an artist works with paint or with tissue and thread. Or maybe another metaphor is more to the point: I have treated my materials in the way chemists do when faced with a mixed liquid. They distil it in order to separate out the various components. In a similar way, I have separated out 'good care' from messy practices. In real life, good care co-exists with other logics as well as with neglect and errors. Here, I have left out such noise in order to distil a 'pure' form out of mixed events.[20] Something coherent, something that could, for as long as it lasts, indeed be called a *logic*. The logic of care – that this book seeks to articulate.

That I use the treatment of, and life with, diabetes in order to articulate the logic of care, has some advantages.[21] Most important, it means that this logic cannot be cast as a pre-modern 'care remnant' in an otherwise modern world. There is nothing nostalgic about diabetes care. As an informant put it: 'Since the moment I have diabetes, the nineteenth century is no longer my favourite period.' People with diabetes (most notably people with type 1 diabetes) depend on modern technologies for their survival. They die quickly without industrially manufactured insulin, and the industrial manufacturing of insulin only began in the late 1920s.[22] That without injectable insulin diabetes is a lethal disease also implies that 'the treatment of' and 'life with' diabetes are not two separate things. Although treatment may take a variety of forms, that allow for different kinds of life, without treatment there is no life. Thus, this case makes it difficult to romantically distrust all technology or to discard 'medicalisation' in general. It also fits my purposes that people with diabetes are as able (or unable) to choose as their neighbours. The disease affects people of all backgrounds and ways of life and is not a 'mental' matter. Thus, if 'choice' does not fit their situation, this is due to this situation rather than to them. What is more: diabetes is a chronic disease and (so far) treatment does not lead to a cure. This implies that what treatment might lead to instead, is overtly attended to in treatment practices. Thus, it can be studied. Overall, studying diabetes care is not too difficult. There is a lot of pain and suffering in diabetes outpatient clinics, and yet this was rarely so acute and overwhelming that I, who had little to offer, felt that I was asking too much of my informants. It was also easy to find people with diabetes willing to be interviewed and most of them had a lot to tell. Finally, I was lucky with the doctors and nurses in the hospital where I carried out my field work. They allowed me to keep a close, critical eye on their work, were open to my questions, and (despite the inevitable noise and messiness) taught me a great deal about 'good care'.

The book

In this book you will not find sentences such as: 'We cannot imagine what it must be like to have a chronic disease.' Sentences like that are nasty. They do not state explicitly that author and reader are in good health, but they imply it all the same. That is not what I am after. On the contrary, I want to avoid unmarked normality. To presume that you and I are healthy would go against the soul of what I seek to say. Within the logic of choice 'disease' is a strange exception, it has nothing to do with 'us', while the logic of care starts out from the fleshiness and fragility of life. I hold that dear. Indeed, in articulating the logic of care I seek to contribute to theoretical repertoires that no longer marginalise, but face disease. As a part of this, it is good to underline that 'patient' and 'philosopher' are by no means mutually exclusive categories. 'I' am not immortal or immune to disease. And your normality, dear reader, is not presupposed here either. Instead, I will use all my rhetorical skills to seduce you – whatever your current diagnosis – to take up the patient's position while you read. The unspecified 'you' in this book, tends to be someone with diabetes. Whether or not you happen to have that disease, I kindly invite you to imagine yourself involved in the situations described. As a patient.

A short overview. The logic of care will be outlined here in a comparison with the logic of choice. In chapter 2 this is, more particularly, the version of the logic of choice that informs the market. In a market, people are interpellated as customers who choose a product to their liking. This product is then handed from seller to buyer in a transaction. Here, the market will be exemplified by an advertisement for a blood sugar monitor. I will analyse this advertisement and compare it with what happens in a purified version of the consulting rooms of the diabetes clinic of hospital Z. Here, professionals appear not to hand over a product to their patients, who, after opting for it, have nothing left to do. Instead, professionals and patients jointly act and act again. Rather than engaging in a transaction, they interact, shifting the action around so as to best accommodate the exigencies of the disease with the habits, requirements and possibilities of daily life. Care is not a limited product, but an ongoing process. ⁄

Chapter 3 starts out from the civic version of the logic of choice. In a democratic state, people are interpellated as citizens who govern themselves and one another. If this model is introduced into health care, and patients are called upon to overturn the dominance of their doctors and emancipate themselves, something is lost. For citizens, or so I will argue while drawing on the tradition of political philosophy, are defined by their ability to control their bodies. However, bodies with a disease are impossible to control: we may take care of them, but they remain unpredictable, erratic. Thus patients may only hope to be citizens in as far as they are healthy. Only their healthy part stands a chance of emancipation. I propose that *patientism* (in analogy with feminism) would do well to not submit to 'normality'. It might do better to explore the way in which the logic of care meticulously attends to the unpredictabilities of bodies with a disease. Caring, or so it appears, is a matter of attuning to, respecting, nourishing and even enjoying mortal bodies.

Chapter 4 deals with professionalism. The ideal of patient choice presupposes professionals who limit themselves to presenting facts and using instruments. In the linear unfolding of a consultation, a professional is supposed to give information, after which the patient can assess his or her values and come to a decision. Only then is it possible to act. However, care practices tend not to be linear at all. Facts do not precede decisions and activities, but depend on what is hoped for and on what can be done. Deciding to do something is rarely enough to actually achieve it. And techniques do more than just serve their function – they have an array of effects, some of which are unexpected. Thus, caring is a question of 'doctoring': of tinkering with bodies, technologies and knowledge – and with people, too.

Chapter 5 moves on to examine how people relate to each other. The logic of choice assumes that we are separate individuals who form a collective when we are added together. In the logic of care by contrast, we do not start out as individuals, but always belong to collectives already – and not just a single one, but a lot of them. The wholes of which we are a part may be named and delineated in various ways. One of the requirements of good care is that such categories are crafted wisely. But how? This is a question that emerges in care practices time and again. Categories are not given once and for all, but need to be made and adapted. They need to be outlined in such a way that they contribute to good care. For whom? This is a difficult question in the logic of care, because care for a population is not just a sum total of the care of and for a lot of individuals. Individuals and collectives require different kinds of care.

In Chapter 6 the lines of my argument come together. The first topic of the chapter is the place the logic of choice and the logic of care accord to questions of morality – or should I say ethics? What, I will more particularly ask, is a moral act? Next, the question as to whether patients need to be freed from passivity is taken up again, for by this point it has become possible to give a better characterisation of the 'active patient'. Following this I touch upon what it might mean to improve health care on its own terms. And then, finally and briefly, I consider what the logic of care might have to offer outside health-care settings. Where else might we want to serve the good life while attending to the viscous reality of erratic, fleshly, mortal bodies?

2   Customer or patient?

The logic of care and the logic of choice each come in several versions. This chapter starts out from choice in its market form and uses this as a point of contrast to the specificities of care.[1] When the language of the market is mobilised, patients are referred to as 'customers'. They buy their care in exchange for money. This implies that patients do not need to feel gratitude for the care they receive, which they might feel obliged to if care were a gift. Instead, the language of the market makes it possible to say that patients are entitled to value for money, and that health care should follow patient demand instead of being supply-driven. The logic of choice suggests that, if supply were indeed to follow demand, care would – at long last – be guided by patients. But will patients really be better off when they are transformed into customers? This is the question I will explore in this chapter. I will not address all aspects of marketisation. Even if I talk about 'the market', the complex issue of how to best finance health care will be bracketed. As will be the role of insurance companies. I will not consider the effects of various combinations of state regulation and market ordering for how professionals end up working. I will also skip questions about the lessons managers of health-care institutions might learn from banks, shops and hotels (how to improve organisational routines, cluster appointments on a single day, make visiting hours more flexible, etc.). Instead I will focus on what happens inside the consulting room. Are patients in a consulting room indeed customers who are eager to buy something? Or is something else going on behind these closed doors?

In order to tackle these questions, I want to present you with an image. I came across this image in *Diabc*, a Dutch monthly magazine for people with diabetes. It was not part of the editorial contents, but

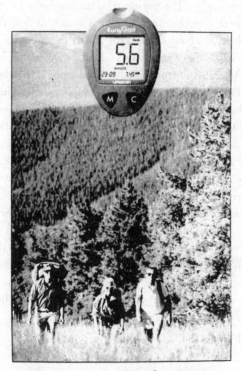

LIFESCAN

a Johnson & Johnson company

Euro*Flash*

perfect in vorm

an advertisement. And it caught my eye. The company that placed the advertisement kindly gave me permission to use it for critical analysis, for which I am grateful. (But for good order I cut off their contact information.) It is a beautiful image, look:

Beautiful young people, walking in the mountains. The blood sugar monitor that hangs above them, larger than life, is beautiful as well. The blue *EuroFlash* is perfect in shape and in perfect shape (the Dutch 'perfect in vorm', printed below the picture, suggests both of these simultaneously). The person who has just used the monitor is also doing well, for the device gives a result of 5.6 (mmol/l).[2] Experts (and the readers of *Diabc*, for whom this advert is intended, are experts) know that this is an excellent blood sugar level. All in all, as we would expect from an advertisement, positive associations abound. In this way LifeScan tries to attract customers. The company wants to sell the *EuroFlash* not for the direct profits, but because each time a potential customer measures her blood sugar levels, she will need a test strip. Such test strips cost around €1 each and are device-specific. The *EuroFlash* test strips can only be used in the *EuroFlash*. A lot of money is involved in this market.[3] However, I am neither concerned with money here, nor with the advantages and disadvantages of this particular blood sugar monitor compared with others. Instead, my question is what happens when a company addresses patients as customers. What happens to disease? And how does this differ from what goes on in a consulting room? In order to answer this question, I will compare the blood sugar monitor that figures in the advertisement above with the blood sugar monitor that appears in the consulting rooms of diabetes nurses and diabetes physicians in the outpatient clinic of hospital Z.

Product or process

Advertisements do not force anything upon potential customers. Instead they offer a choice. Here it is, the *EuroFlash*, do you want it? The suggestion is that as a customer you are made active rather than passive. It is up to you. Markets are places where supply adapts to demand. This means that customers exercise discretion: they control the demand. Their demand will not be questioned: customers are always right.[4] However, being in charge can be difficult. You must call the shots, but how? Indeed, this is a common theme in criticisms of marketisation: as patient-customers we are left alone. There you are, at home, with your *Diabc*. The magazine is packed with adverts for highly recommended blood sugar monitors. Which one to choose? Within health care, choosing a suitable blood sugar monitor has by tradition been a task of the diabetes nurse. She is aware that young people prefer to have a device that is easy to carry around and that looks attractive, while such designer devices do not suit older people, since their components are too small to handle. A diabetes nurse thinks about the length of time that passes between the moment you insert a test strip into the device and the moment when the results appear. She checks whether or not the display is easy to read. If the device has an advantage or a disadvantage she has failed to notice, she quickly learns about it from her patients. Professionals collect patient experiences and pass them on from one person to the next.

Is this the difference between the logic of choice and that of care: that on the market customers can make active choices but have to do so on their own, while care provides patients with an instrument that is tailored to their needs, but gives them no say in the matter? No, it is more complex than this. For in the consulting room, nurses relate to their patients. 'What is important to you?' they ask with several measuring devices laid out on the table, 'What do you want?' At the same time, patient-customers are not necessarily on their own. They may organise themselves. Like other customers, patients can have their products tested or share their experiences without professional go-betweens. They can collectively acquire detailed knowledge of the niche market for the devices tailored to their needs. Websites and patient magazines may gradually collect all the relevant information. This is one of the creative innovations made possible by the market: as organised consumers, patients help each other to choose.

However, choosing a particular blood sugar monitor is not enough. Somehow you have to learn how to use your new machine. Here the diabetes nurse tends to make her appearance again. 'Look Mrs Jansen, you must prick with this thing, this needle. Hold it like this. Yes, that's right. And now prick here, on the side of your fingertip, never on the top, but on the side. Right, there. Would you like to try it yourself now, or shall I do it for you first, so you can feel it? It doesn't hurt, don't worry.' And so on. How to squeeze out the drop of blood and catch it on the test strip; how to place the test strip in the device; how to record the results in the notebook; how to respond to those results. When advertisements present a blood sugar monitor as an independent product, this learning process is hidden. This does not particularly trouble potential *EuroFlash* customers who read *Diabc:* their diabetes nurse explained how to use a monitor a long time ago. But even so there is something troubling about presenting a blood sugar monitor as a separate sellable product, disentangled from the care process in which it is embedded. So what is that?

One might say that the *EuroFlash* advert tries to sell a device without mentioning the support necessary in using it. But *this* is not a problem inherent to the market. Instead it is an historical coincidence that grows out of the way health care is currently organised. LifeScan has to present the *EuroFlash* as a separate product to its potential customers because it finds itself in a position where it can put 'things' in a market much more easily than the 'services' of nurses. The latter are already organised in another way. However, over recent decades the economy has amply demonstrated that services can perfectly well be sold commercially. Indeed, not only are services lucrative products in their own right, but many goods sell a lot better if they come with the necessary service attached. It is quite likely that, had the profession not existed already, LifeScan and its competitors would have invented the diabetes nurse. As things stand, these companies willingly subsidise courses and other meetings for diabetes nurses, since this helps to strengthen the service on which their products depend.

No, if the work of diabetes nurses is undervalued, this is not the market's fault. All sorts of things can be traded in markets: devices, skills training, and even kindness and attention. Customers appreciate kindness and attention. So the point is not that the market leads to cold and distanced relations, not at all. What it does, however, is draw a limit. The market requires that some product (device, plus skills training, plus kindness and attention) is delineated as the product on offer. A lot may be included in this product, but what is on offer and what it is not has to be specified.[5] Then, or so the logic of choice has it, you may choose it, or not. This is a crucial difference with the logic of care. Care is a process: it does not have clear boundaries. It is open-ended. This is not a matter of size; it does not mean that a care process is larger, more encompassing, than the devices

while, often no more than once every few months, just before their regular check-up. The technician would take a blood sample and get it measured, and the physician would adjust the daily dose or doses of insulin if this was necessary. You might also, in exceptional cases, go to the lab several times a day for a single day or a few days in a row. Or you might be admitted to the hospital for detailed monitoring. But these were exceptions. Once your insulin dose was readjusted your blood sugar might not be measured for quite a while. So measuring one's own blood sugar levels regularly is not necessary for immediate survival. Instead, it serves another purpose: it makes it possible to fine-tune the amount of insulin to be injected. If patients measure their own blood sugar levels, they can do so a lot more often than laboratory technicians. This means that physicians are better able to adjust the doses they prescribe, and patients themselves may also decide to inject a bit more or less depending on the current state of their bodies. With such fine-tuned dosing, care gets better.

This means care may sometimes improve even when professionals are supplying less 'product' and patients are doing more work themselves. The implication is not that good care equals neglect. What matters in the logic of care is the outcome, the result. Who takes on which task follows from this. The technician may measure your blood sugar for you or you may measure your blood sugar yourself, as long as the joint efforts lead to improvement. To complicate things, it is not always clear what to count as 'improvement'. Traditionally, health was the ultimate goal of health care. These days it rarely is. In chronic diseases health is beyond reach, and it has been replaced by the ideal of a 'good life'. But what counts as a 'good life' is neither clear nor fixed. Aiming for a long and happy life might sound nice, but it is often necessary to juggle between 'long' and 'happy'. Despite these complexities, in one way or another, unstable blood sugar levels are bad. Thus, it is good care to try to figure out how to stabilise blood sugar levels. This is not to say that good care leads to stable blood sugar levels: trying does not guarantee success. Within the logic of care, therefore, it is not a surprise if blood sugar levels remain unstable even though the entire care team does its best. That is how it is, diseased bodies are unpredictable. It follows from this unpredictability that care is not a well-delineated product, but an open-ended process. Try, adjust, try again. In dealing with a disease that is chronic, the care process is chronic, too. It only ends the day you die.

Thus, the problem with the logic of choice is not that the market abandons people: consumers can help each other with their choices and they may buy as much kindness and attention as they can afford. However, and this is my point, in one way or another a market requires that the product that changes hands in a transaction be clearly defined. It must have a beginning and an end. In the logic of care, by contrast, care is an interactive, open-ended process that may be shaped and reshaped depending on its results. This difference is irreducible. It implies that a care process may improve even though less product is being supplied. What counts is whether or not the results are better. More complicated still: even though care is result-oriented, it is not necessarily bad when 'health' and a 'good life' remain out of reach. Some diseases can never be cured, some problems keep on shifting. Even if good care strives after good results, the quality of care cannot be deduced from its results. Instead, what characterises good care is a calm, persistent but forgiving effort to improve the situation of a patient, or to keep this from deteriorating.

Target group or team member

When I write to Johnson & Johnson, the holding company of Life-Scan, to ask permission to use their advertisement, I not only receive the required permission, but a visitor as well. A friendly young woman from the marketing department, involved in her work, concerned about her customers, eager to learn from my criticism. What exactly is my point, she asks. Why am I uncomfortable with this advert? I don't quite know yet, so I tell her the story of an elderly couple we interviewed. (Leaving out clues that might have identified them — just as I do throughout this book.) The husband has diabetes and they no longer go on holiday because it takes too much effort. The tour bus will arrive at the hotel at eight o'clock in the evening, but *he* is used to having his dinner at five-thirty. How to handle this? The next day the evening meal is at seven and, what is more, the evening coffee comes with cake. Should he eat this or not? It is too complicated. Holiday rudely disrupts daily routines. Advertisements like yours, I tell my guest, stand in stark contrast with such stories. They suggest that, if you use the *EuroFlash*, anything is possible, it is in perfect shape. If you cannot walk in the mountains despite it, you have only yourself to blame.

The marketing manager listens attentively. Well, yes, she says, but the people you talk about now belong to a different target group. Look, and she pulls out another advert, this is what we offer to them. Her picture shows a slightly simpler blood sugar monitor and a man in a striped polo shirt, who does not seem too ambitious either. The finger he holds ready for pricking is magnified. Pricking blood is made to appear an entirely practical task, no promises (of mountain walks or other wonders) attached. The simpler monitor is presented as a purely functional tool. A market, or so my guest tells me, consists of different target groups. Some people may be unable to go on holiday, or to the mountains, and of course we do not ask them to do so. For them we make simple devices. Others, however, want freedom. They want to go abroad, visit cities, enjoy holidays, have novel experiences, and indeed, walk in the mountains. These may be better-educated people, but this is not necessarily so. What is crucial is that they understand the intricacies of the disease and are willing to make an effort. 'People like you and me,' she says. They form a separate target group. For them we have developed the *EuroFlash* and the advertisement of young people eagerly walking.

In order to put a product on the market, it is important to identify its target group. My visitor presents me with a carefully designed sheet. This shows the four relevant target groups for blood sugar monitors: those who know a lot and want a lot; those who know a lot but want little; those who know little but still want a lot; and finally those who both know little and want little. In the course of my research, I will come across a number of more or less similar fourfold divisions. For example, at a conference with the telling title 'Customers in Careland', a speaker from the Rabobank, a Dutch banking group, says that the bank divides potential customers according to the type of relationships they engage in: those looking for independence, those looking for harmony, those looking for certainty, and those looking for control.[6] From behind his podium, pointing at the audience, he adds: 'You, in the health-care world, you should also separate your customers out into target groups.' He thinks it is about time that self-satisfied health-care professionals understood that different groups of people want different things from them.

But should 'we in the health-care world' really begin to divide people into target groups? This does not fit with the logic of care. The marketing manager of Johnson & Johnson helped me to articulate why not, when she said that the target group for the mountain walk advertisement was 'people like you and me'. An expression like this assumes that 'people like you and me', clever and able, have no problem in organising mountain walks, even though other people might find this difficult. But it is not so easy. As it happens, on the day we spoke, I was grateful that *she* had come to visit *me*. I was not well at all. Thus, I was just about capable of talking with her, but would not have had the energy to travel to her office. Going for a walk in the mountains, no matter how attractive, was even further beyond my capabilities. I did not belong to her category 'you and me'.[7] Care professionals are not surprised by such things. They do not make categories based on a sociological marker or two. Instead, at least if they give good care, they inquire into the specific situation of a specific person. 'How are you?' a good professional might have asked me. 'Are you unable to travel even for an hour or two? That must be hard on you.' Care makes space for what is *not* possible. Everyone can come to a consulting room and complain (to an appropriate degree, that is). Even people 'like you and me'.

In the logic of care fragility is taken to be a part of life. But care professionals not only accept that sooner or later everyone may need help, they also refuse to give up on anyone. Salespeople do. A group of people to whom nothing can be sold stops being a 'target' group. People who 'know nothing and want nothing' will not buy a blood sugar monitor and, if they get one for free, they will not use it. In a market this means that it is a bad investment to keep targeting them. The logic of care, by contrast, does not start out from what people know or want but from what they need. Thus caring professionals do not abandon their patients, but keep on trying. As a physician puts it, while we are waiting in the consulting room: 'We expect nothing much from the next patient. I no longer push him, nor does Maria (the diabetes nurse). There is no point. He just doesn't take proper care of himself. But fortunately he regularly comes for his check-ups, so we keep things going.' Doctor and nurse no longer press this patient, but still receive him with a typical clinical mixture of friendliness and severity. They listen to his stories and answer his questions. ('What should I do if I have just a small temperature? Should I stay home or go to work?' the patient asks. 'Don't take your temperature,' replies the doctor.) I do not want to romanticise what happens in consulting rooms when professionals 'keep things going'.

But even in moments that leave a lot to be desired, health-care professionals do not write people off as bad investments.

In the market variant of the logic of choice customers are divided
into target groups. This makes it possible to match products to their
potential buyers and advertise them effectively. Those who want
freedom are promised freedom; those who do not, are presented
with something simpler; and those who cannot be tempted to buy
anything at all are left in peace. In the logic of care it is different. The
point is not that health-care practices abstain from categorising
people. A lot depends on categories such as 'type 1 diabetes' and
'type 2 diabetes': the organisation of outpatient clinics; assembling
groups of patients together for courses and patient support groups;
arranging payments; conducting scientific research. Diagnostic categories, however, are not based on what people are likely to want,
but on what they might need. What is more, in the day-to-day practice of care these categories fall apart. Hands-on care is concerned
with the specific problems of specific individuals in specific circumstances. The art of care is to figure out how various actors (professionals, medication, machines, the person with a disease and others
concerned) might best collaborate in order to improve, or stabilise, a
person's situation. What to do and how to share the doing? In the
logic of care, patients are not a target group, but crucial members of
the care team.[8]

Dreams or support

Maybe some people are not able to go on holiday, or so the marketing manager of Johnson & Johnson says, but others want freedom. In
saying this, she not only distinguishes between groups of people, but
also suggests that 'what people want' is a given. It is the demand to
which producers/sellers need to target their supply. This is the language of neo-classical economics, in which customers are people who
make rational choices and stick to them. However, at the same time,
my guest is responsible for marketing Johnson & Johnson's blood
sugar monitors. Thus she went to an advertising agency and ordered
two advertisements: one for the simple monitor her company produces and another for the *EuroFlash*. The first had to evoke ease, efficiency and simplicity; the second was meant to appeal to 'people
who want freedom'. What might seduce them into thinking that the

EuroFlash will bring such freedom? In contrast with neo-classical economists, advertising agencies are not at all inclined to treat 'demand' as something that is given. For them 'what people want' is not a rational phenomenon, they try to create demand. Not with arguments, but through seduction.

Three young people walking in the mountains: it looks just great. The *EuroFlash* capitalises on the desire of potential customers to be able to go out and walk. This walking has little to do with putting one foot in front of the other; getting into a rhythm; sweating; or enjoying the wandering.[9] What is at stake instead is the ability to walk, to go wherever you might want to go. This advert appeals (as it was meant to do) to the desires of 'people who want freedom'. But it is nourishing these desires at the same time. Look at the photo again. It shows people walking in the mountains, but what is represented is not so much walking, as freedom. The freedom to escape from the pressures of modern life into the otherness of nature. The freedom to go where the birds go and to forget about diabetes. This is a common advertising strategy. An attractive situation that can be captured in an image represents something else, a higher good, an ideal beyond it. Meanwhile the situation depicted is stripped of its specificity. No wonder this advertisement caught my eye: I love walking. I am suspicious of the suggestion that freedom (forever out of reach) is more important than walking.

The logic of care does not similarly exploit desires. Granted, if walking happens to be mentioned in the consulting room, it is unlikely that this is to celebrate it 'for its own sake'. Some professionals may be walkers themselves; others will empathise with whatever their patients happen to be keen about. But the clinically relevant characteristic of walking, the one that is first and foremost relevant in the consulting room, is that it is a way of getting exercise. It increases your overall fitness, stimulates the circulation, and only rarely leads to accidents. For these reasons a diabetes nurse is likely to encourage walking. Yes, she will nod, walking, very good. And then she will warn you to carry enough food with you on a walk, because when exercising muscles burn sugar and your blood sugar level is likely to drop. Don't just refrain from injecting insulin, for your cells will need both food and insulin to have enough sugar to burn. And beware: diabetes tends to slow the healing of small wounds on your feet. So you should wear good shoes and socks in order to protect your feet, says the nurse. Good shoes and socks are not attractive, they are necessary. The difference in register is striking. In the consulting room of a diabetes nurse walking does not call up a dream, but calls rather for practicalities. It is not associated with freedom, but with socks.

Conversations in the consulting room of a diabetes nurse tend to concentrate on topics like socks. They focus on the endless practical details of daily life that are mysteriously absent from the *EuroFlash* advertisement. For while this enticing image presents us with a promise of freedom, it hides everything that users of blood sugar monitors actually need to do in order to be able to walk in the mountains. Blood sugar monitors do not work on their own, they depend on the activities of their users. Stop walking, sit down somewhere, clean your fingers. (Where did that tissue go?) Prick your finger, catch the drop of blood on the test strip, put the strip into the machine. Wait, read the number. Respond to it. And measuring your blood sugar levels is not enough. In order to walk in the mountains, you need to do a lot more. Keep your insulin cool; take enough food with you; eat on time, enough but not too much. Rest when you are tired, even if the others want to carry on walking. Carefully manage your dealings with your companions. 'Shouldn't you eat something now?' 'Let me be.' But if your blood sugar level becomes too low, one of them will have to inject you with glucagon in order to get you out of your coma.

Dealing with your own unpredictable blood sugar levels is not attractive. In health care nobody suggests that it is. Instead, it is sensible to do all these things. Professionals who encourage patients to take care of themselves appeal to their patients' minds, not their desires. They explain that taking good care of yourself, no matter how difficult it may be, is likely to postpone the nasty complications of diabetes. Statistics show that people with badly regulated blood sugar levels tend to suffer more and sooner from blindness, clogged-up arteries, and loss of sensation in their limbs. Such threatening prospects make it advisable to try and control your blood sugar levels. Care is not attractive. Let me underline this, even good care is not attractive. If only because as a patient you cannot just buy it, as if it were a product for passive consumption. Instead you have to engage actively in care, painfully, enduringly, and as a prominent member of the care team. That is demanding. And yet you may take these demands on board, because suffering from complications is likely to be a lot nastier.

Chronic diseases make life even more difficult than it already is. The logic of care is attuned to that difficulty and concludes from it that patients deserve support (advice, encouragement, consolation). However, offering support is not the same thing as doing what patients want. It does not mean going along with them. While the market fuels the desires that it mobilises (such as the desire for freedom), care seeks moderation. Balance is the magic word. 'You don't really want an early death, do you? Or to go blind?' says a doctor severely to a woman who is taking good care of her children, her husband, her job, and her ideals, but not of her blood sugar levels. In this somewhat rough way he tries to make her realise how important it is for her to take better care of herself. But trying too hard to take care of yourself is not good either. 'The worst people are those who think they can stay below 10 (mmol/l) all the time. Help, doctor, I once had a blood sugar level of 11, they say to me. Yes, of course you have a blood sugar level of 11 once in while. What else would you expect?' Doctors do not go along with people who are too obsessive in their attempts at self-control. Instead they counter the worries of such people with some version of: 'Come on, these things happen, let it go.' Fighting against the unpredictability that is inherent to life with a disease only leads to more misery. It is not a sensible thing to do.

Thus, in care practices our minds are called upon, not our desires. But this does not lead to rationalism. Our desires may not be rational, but, or so the logic of care has it, neither are our minds. Instead, they are full of gaps, contradictions and obsessions. Caring professionals therefore seek to cultivate our minds. They convey insights, ask probing questions, or try to reassure us. And in doing so, they try not just to reflect back what we thought already. In the hope of making us more balanced, they give counterbalance. They encourage us to take good care of ourselves, without feeding the illusion of control. Unpleasant surprises are to be expected. On advertisements for blood sugar monitors, there is no room for unpleasant surprises. Marketing is a matter of seduction. Look! Imagine yourself walking in the mountains! Thanks to our wonderful blood sugar monitor! That walking in the mountains might also go wrong is never mentioned. Anyway, the *EuroFlash* cannot be blamed for troubles: maybe you are the one who fails? No, this is not mentioned either. But on the market such fears are evoked, in all of us, including you and me. There is nobody to contradict them. In good care practices, by contrast, the fear of failure is explicitly addressed. A caring professional reminds you that, no matter what statistics may promise, everything is erratic, from diseases, to mountains, machines, friends and blood sugar levels. Unpredictable. Do your best, but if this turns out not to be good enough, let go. Don't take the world on your shoulders.

Hoping for health or living with disease

The advertisement for the *EuroFlash* mobilises the desire to be free in order to sell blood sugar monitors to 'people who want freedom'. It plays with other desires as well. The desire to walk, to be young, to have friends. And the desire to be healthy. Look at the advertisement again: it does not show test strips; there is no blood; nothing messy, nothing that speaks of disease. The well-designed blood sugar monitor looks like any 'normal' tool, a walking pole for instance, that also helps you to walk in the mountains. Walking itself also evokes associations with 'health'. And with a blood sugar level of 5.6 (mmol/l), the walker who has just used the *EuroFlash* is in perfect shape. Who, by the way, is the user of the *EuroFlash* in the advertisement? It is impossible to tell. The image shows three equally vital and energetic walkers.[10] So even though it is never explicitly stated that the *EuroFlash* will bring health, health is visible in this image. Absent present, it is represented in various ways.[11]

Many people with diabetes do not feel ill. Nor should they be reduced to their disease: there is more to life than one's diagnoses. However, at present diabetes (and certainly type 1) is a chronic disease that cannot be cured and does not go away. This means that appealing to the desire for health in an advertisement for a blood sugar monitor is a remarkable way of playing with desires. It might well make potential buyers more enthusiastic than the worrying tone of health-care counselling. Instead of rubbing patients' noses in the miseries of long-time complications and encouraging them to sensibly take proper care of themselves, they are seduced into dreaming of wonderful things: walking, freedom, health! But inciting such dreams makes it possible to keep on selling goods for as long as the customers can pay. There are, after all, no limits to the desire for health among people with chronic disease.[12]

Good care strives for improvement while simultaneously respecting the erratic character of disease. Let us revisit the scene in which the diabetes nurse explains to Mrs Jansen how to prick for blood. This scene is typical of the way care tries to tame disease without denying it. 'You should hold it like this, yes, very good. And then you prick here, on the side of your fingertip, never on the top, but on the side. There it is.' Mrs Jansen learns how to measure her own blood sugar levels in order to avoid, or at least to postpone, the complications of diabetes. One of these complications is blindness. Measuring blood sugar levels is meant to prevent blindness. But from day one, Mrs Jansen learns not to prick the top of her fingertip, but its side. The reason for this is that people who do go blind despite their best efforts will need the tops of their fingertips in order to feel the world around them. Thus at the very moment when one learns how to prick, there is hope of health as well as acceptance of disease. You learn how to prick so that you may stay as healthy as possible. But you respect the fact that the reality of disease is erratic by practically anticipating the complications, blindness included, that may occur even so.

In the logic of care promising something too good to be true is a professional sin. Tempting, perhaps, but wrong. 'It is difficult,' confesses a physician in an interview. 'You have to ask people to do something that is incredibly difficult to do: to watch over themselves the whole time, to continuously do their very best to keep their blood sugars down. This is for later, you add, because they may feel fine with a blood sugar of 12 or 15, higher even. Then they see someone in the waiting room whose leg has been amputated. This is frightening. Very much so. So they ask me: "Doctor, if I try really hard, is this not going happen to me?" But I cannot promise anything. You never know. It may well happen to them.' Diseases are erratic, so good doctors do not make promises. There is only one certainty: in the end, you die. The moment will be different for each of us, but that it will come is certain. When no more interventions work, your doctor may say: I am sorry, but there is nothing more I can do for you. And even if your desire for life has not left you, from that moment onwards you may be offered support and sympathy, but heroic actions are abandoned.[13] In the logic of care there is a limit to activism. This is another irreducible difference: on a market almost anything may be traded, but there is nothing to limit futile transactions. How to say 'there is nothing I can do for you' on a market? 'No' is hard to sell.

Actors who let go

The logic of choice refers to people seeking help as 'customers' instead of using the old term 'patients', that is etymologically related to 'passive'. It addresses us as 'customers in careland'. Like other customers, those with diabetes are invited to enter the market to buy products that they find attractive: insulin, monitors, attention. Within the logic of care, by contrast, people who seek help are called 'patients' for good reasons: they suffer. Patients have a disease that they did not choose to have. But this does not imply that the logic of care makes patients passive. Instead, care activities move between doctors, nurses, machines, drugs, needles and so on, while patients have to do a lot as well. They have to eat and drink, inject, measure and/or engage in exercise. They care.

When it calls patients 'customers' the logic of choice opens up splendid panoramic views. From the top of the mountain you see no suffering. The language of the market contains only positive terms. Products for sale are attractive. Tellingly and non-neutrally, they are called 'goods'. The logic of care, by contrast, starts out from something negative: you would prefer not to have diabetes. And if you do, you will never be healthy again. But the fact that health is out of reach does not mean that you should give up. The active patient that the logic of care tries to make of us is a flexible, resilient actor who, by caring, strives after as much health as her disease allows. What the results of the joint activities of a care team turn out to be is uncertain. Diseases are unpredictable. The art of care, therefore, is to act without seeking to control. To persist while letting go. That is care: wherever you are, if you need to, you sit down, prick the side of your fingertip, squeeze out some blood, put the test strip into the blood sugar monitor, and wait for the results to appear on the screen.

must be open to their professionals about everything that is relevant to their disease. Professionals, in turn, have to respect the fact that it is the patient who actively commissioned their help. Thus, in the Netherlands (and in most other Western countries) professionals are now under the legal obligation to allow their patients to decide what will happen in the course of a diagnostic and treatment trajectory. Professionals must provide their patients with information and then ask about what they want. They may only act once patients have given their explicit consent and, if there are different options, patients should have the legal right to choose between these.

In the civic version of the logic of choice professionals in the consulting room are not considered to be selling their patients a product. Instead, the relationship is moulded in the form of a contract. This contract does away with medical authority: it respects doctors (as well as other health professionals) and patients as equals. They have different roles, the contract demands different things of each, but they are both civic actors. How, you may wonder, might anyone seriously doubt that this is a good thing? Surely your author is not going to advocate a return to patriarchal authority? And indeed, that is not what I am after. And yet in this chapter I will argue that figuring as a citizen in the consulting room is not as wonderful as it may seem to be. This is not because, when it comes to it, the doctor (nurse, dietician, physical therapist, etc.) knows best. If I question the civic version of the logic of choice, my aim is not to frustrate the emancipation of patients. Instead, I would like to go beyond it.

Emancipation may well be an improvement over oppression, but at the same time it is a rather limited ideal. This is a lesson from the women's movement: striving for equality between 'women' and 'men' meant that women were 'allowed' to become just like men – insofar as this is practically possible. But, however nice this may sound, it implies that 'men' remain the standard. What is more: the limits to what is 'practically possible' work out in such a way that, when it comes to it, women will never be 'just like men'. Thus, in the women's movement emancipation has been supplemented with another strategy: that of feminism. Instead of moving the figures around, feminism interferes with the categories. It questions the very definitions of 'woman' and 'man', it interferes with the masculine standard. My suggestion is that the patient movement might imagine doing something similar. By analogy with feminism, we might call it *patientism* – even though this is not a wonderful word. (Please, reader, come up with a better one!) The point is this: if patients in the consulting room are 'allowed' to become citizens insofar as this is practically possible, citizenship is established as the standard. At first, this may seem fine. Citizens, after all, are not bossed around by patriarchal rulers. Their contract stipulates that they are masters of their own lives. However, on closer examination something seems to be missing. By definition, citizens are not troubled by their bodies. But patients are.[2]

Unlike the previous chapter, where I had an advertisement to take apart, this chapter does not use a single emblematic patient-citizen as a point of contrast for stories from the consulting room. Instead, as my concern is with the fact that 'by definition, citizens are not troubled by their bodies', I will explore the *definition* of the citizen. As the term 'citizen' was gradually and variably framed in the course of the history of Western political theory, I will make a few excursions into this history. I will present you with the (very rough!) outlines of three variants of the 'citizen' that, while first delineated a long time ago, still resonate in our present understanding. What they have in common is that their bodies never interfere with their plans. 'By definition' a citizen is someone who controls his body, who tames it, or who escapes from it. 'Citizens' owe the ability to make their own choices to the silence of their organs.[3] But this implies that you can only be a citizen in as far as your body can be controlled, tamed or transcended. Diseases interfere with this. Thus patient-citizens have to bracket a part of what they are. As a patient, you may only hope to be a citizen with your healthy part. Never completely, never as a whole.

In the civic version of the logic of choice bodies have to be subjugated. And however nice emancipation may sound, this subjugation of the body is quite a price for patients to pay. Might it not be possible for patients to be taken seriously, disease and all? That is what *patientism* is about. It does not seek equality between 'patients' and 'healthy people', but tries to establish living with a disease, rather than 'normality', as the standard. It stresses that it is our common condition that from dust we come and to dust we shall return. While citizenship requires us to control our bodies, to silence them, or to discard them, *patientism* seeks ways to be kind to our bodies, to allow them to exist, and even to cherish them. Where to find repertoires for doing so? It may sound strange to those who believe that patriarchal professionals are in the business of oppressing patients, but suitable repertoires for attending to bodies can be found in the consulting room.[4] A lot of what is going on there needs to be improved. *Patientism* still has a long way to go. But it is likely to learn more from the care given in consulting rooms than from the rules and regulations written down in patient laws. To argue this, I will present you with three theoretical framings of the citizen-body and contrast these with snapshot stories of care practices. How does the logic of care attune to fleshly, fragile, mortal bodies?

Control or attentiveness

The first layer of meaning that resonates in the current term 'citizen' comes from Greek political theory, or what has been made of it. The Greek polis was not ruled by tyrants but by an assembly of free men. If an important decision was to be made, these men would gather in the city's public square, the agora. If the city had to be defended against strangers, they would fight. Their ability to act depended on the power of their will and the strength of their muscular bodies.[5] There are still statues left of these strong heroes, the well-honed muscles clearly visible beneath the smoothly polished skin. For Greek citizens, control over their bodies was identical with control over their muscles. Not all muscles, for those of the heart and the intestines move autonomously. But as a Greek citizen, you were supposed to train yourself in order to bring your voluntary muscles under ever better command of your will. In this way you would never become a puppet in someone else's hands – a slave. A free man could control the world in pretty much the same way that he controlled his muscles: from a decisive centre.

In talk about living with diabetes the word 'control' is frequently used for people's attempts to stabilise their blood sugar level from the outside. But that term is misleading, for attending to one's metabolism does not begin to resemble controlling one's muscles. Face it: sugar is being burned in all the cells of a body. This process cannot be steered from a centre. It is not steered from a centre in a body without diabetes, but neither can it be brought under voluntary control from the outside. It depends on far too many variables. It is impossible to control them all: unexpected things always happen. Learning to achieve metabolic balance is therefore not a question of

strengthening one's muscles and hardening one's will, but of learning
to be attentive. In order to live with diabetes, one needs sensitivity
and flexibility. Watch out what goes on and respond. Be adaptable.

As a part of this, you have to relate wisely to your surroundings.
The muscular body of a Greek soldier is sealed off by a skin, but the
metabolic body of a person with diabetes absorbs food and fluids from
the outside, and expels waste. It does not keep all that is foreign to it
outside itself, but exchanges matter with the rest of the world. A
moment ago, the apple was still in the fruit bowl. Now you have
bitten into it, chewed and swallowed it, and started to partially digest
it. A moment ago, the water was still in your glass, now it is being
absorbed in your intestines and thinning your blood, which will
thicken again in your kidneys. The boundaries are not open. The
intestinal lining allows carbohydrates to pass, but it stops bacteria.
Lung parenchyma allows oxygen to enter, but keeps soot particles out.
Urea exits via the kidneys, but protein is not meant to do so. Neither
closed off, nor open, the boundaries of a metabolic body are semi-per-
meable. What passes through them and what does not, cannot be controlled from a single centre. But it has to be attended to and all the
more so if you have diabetes. As a body with diabetes does not silently
regulate its own sugar uptake, you have to actively balance the energy
in your beans, your bread and your apples with the energy you use up
and the amount of insulin you inject. You have to inject insulin.[6]

For Greek free men, eating is something that they do in private.
Women and slaves make their meals. Once their bellies are filled, the
men leave the house again, and join the other men in the agora where
they may publically discuss matters of the city state. For people with
diabetes, by contrast, it is obvious that metabolic affairs are no
private matter. They are always also public in kind. It is not just their
food that comes from elsewhere and that only appears on their table
if it has been grown, transported, bought, cleaned, cooked. They
may do some of these things themselves, but others are done by
others. Family, friends and/or people who earn their living this way.
This goes for all of us. But the metabolism of people with diabetes
also depends on something beyond their skin. In the 1950s, when the
industrial production of insulin was still fairly new, people with diabetes in the Netherlands used to say: 'My pancreas is in Oss.' Oss
was the home town of the Organon factory, which produced their
insulin.

But if one's insulin is produced outside one's body, how does it get inside? If insulin were eaten, it would be broken down in the intestines. Thus it must be injected. Straight through the skin. 'For now, I will inject your insulin for you, Mrs Alzari,' says the nurse. 'Tomorrow it's your turn. Please, have a look now. Look what I do. No, it won't hurt you. Are you scared? Hey, it's done already. That wasn't too bad, was it?' Insulin is injected with a needle. In contrast to the traditional syringes, present-day needles are tiny. The devices to which they are attached are called 'pens' (despite the impressive improvement, this is still a remarkable euphemism). 'At first I used to hide to inject myself,' says Harold Lee. 'But now I no longer do. I don't care where I am. Having a pen makes it easier, since if needs be you go straight through your clothes. So I am in a restaurant and I say: "Guys, I need a shot." Or I don't say anything. I just do my thing.' Pens may be easy to use, but using them remains a hassle. It requires attention. What happens automatically inside bodies without diabetes, requires a lot of work on the outside of bodies with diabetes. Interviewer: 'Do you find it annoying, that pen?' Tanja Trudijn: 'No. No, I don't. Listen, my life depends on it. And I do it so often, I'm used to it. That pen … eh, that is a part of me.' Just as insulin, through being injected, is incorporated into the body, a pen, through being used again and again, is incorporated into the self. This happens more easily with an attractive pen than with one that looks scary. This is why designer pens are an improvement: you can show them off when you are dining in a restaurant. No need to hide that part of you.

A body may be spread out to small towns far away, and a pen may become part of a person. Thus metabolism is not just a physical process. It also offers a model for what it might mean to be an actor. The Greek citizen controls his muscles and movements from a centre and his body is closed off by his skin. If he learns to control himself he will not fall into the hands of his enemies. He will be nobody's slave. Metabolic actors need not fear that they might become a puppet in somebody else's hands: who would be able to hold the strings? Instead, they run another risk: they may burn up and disintegrate. In order to avoid this fate, they have to balance the energy they absorb and the energy they expend very carefully. Staying in metabolic balance does not depend on central control and a forceful will, but on dispersed coordination, inside and beyond the skin. This is what the logic of care is concerned with. Caring is not a matter of control let alone of oppression. It does not involve staying free or making someone else into a slave. Instead, it is a matter of attending to the balances inside, and the flows between, a fragile body and its intricate surroundings.

Tame or nourish

A second figure that resonates in our current term 'citizen' is the bourgeois, a person marked out by being civilised. Control of one's body is again important to this figure, but muscular force is not. Civilised citizens do not need to master their movements, they should tame their passions.[7] Christianity identified passions as lust. It was a sin to act in accordance with one's lusts. A good Christian needed to tame the beast inside. When political philosophers started to define citizens as people who are able to govern themselves, who do not need an overlord, they no longer spoke of 'sin'. However, passions still needed to be tamed. This was because passions cloud our ability to reason. People who are ruled by their passions, or so the reasoning went, are selfish. This implies that they cannot establish the 'common good' and cannot solve conflicts among themselves. They fight. Thus, as long as people are all too passionate, they need an authority above them to end their conflicts. The ability to tame one's passions is a precondition for self-rule: it defines the bourgeois citizen.

At the time when philosophers wrote treatises about the passions, etiquette books were also speaking about controlling the beast inside. Beware, citizens, do not burp, fart, babble drunkenly or wield knives. Leave your weapons at home when you visit public spaces. Only spit in spittoons. In day-to-day practices, bodily behaviour had to be brought under control.[8] The well-tamed body that results is characterised by its apparent absence. There are still traces of such civility today. Take the situation so typical for the celebration of our citizenship: the public meeting. Calmly take your seat. While the meeting lasts, you will not shuffle, fidget, yawn, sleep, scream or scratch yourself. Your body is supposed to be able to postpone its needs for food, beverages and toilet breaks (not to mention sex). Meetings require us to be physically present, but our bodies have to simultaneously absent themselves.

In the consulting room patients describe how difficult this is. It is difficult for everyone, but for people with slightly more demanding bodies meetings are even worse. Henriette Tilstra reports to her physician: 'My new job is going fine. But it's not easy. The content is not the problem, really, but what's hard is being in these meetings that take forever. And then I think I'm getting low, my blood sugars are. And I don't know what to do. I don't like to eat there, on the spot, it would be weird, nobody ever eats during these meetings. Maybe I should just leave, go to the toilet and measure, check if what I feel is right, if I'm really low. But that would be odd too. Nobody does that either. They all stay put. While of course, what I'm really afraid of, is getting a hypo during a meeting. I definitely don't want to be saying weird things in a meeting.' A body with a hypo (that is, with hypoglycaemia, a blood sugar level that is too low) acts wildly. It may say unpleasant, aggressive things, begin to swear. Bystanders may learn to attribute such transgressions to your disease. If so, they may forgive you. But will they still take you seriously a little later, after you have eaten? You cannot tell. Thus hypos are to be avoided during meetings. However, at the same time you are not supposed to do what you need to do in order to ensure this. Civil bodies are to be subjected to the agenda of the meeting. Eating, leaving, measuring blood sugars, none of these are in order.

In the consulting room, by contrast, a body is not a silent but necessary precondition for speech. It is the very entity that speaks. From a physical perspective, speaking is not an easy task. It depends on such things as a mouth that is not too dry, sufficient breath, and a high enough blood sugar level. Such bodily requirements of speech are not given in the order of things. They call for care, sometimes for extra care, and in the consulting room such care is attended to. Thus conversations in the consulting room are not about what is being said at meetings ('the content is not the problem, really'). Instead they are about the physical ability to talk – or to talk sense. Henriette Tilstra and her physician examine how she might best deal with meetings. Maybe it would be better always to eat something before a meeting begins. Maybe Henriette's colleagues should get used to her leaving now and then. Maybe the issue of hypoglycaemia should be made explicit, but then again, maybe not (colleagues may have strange reactions to disease). In the consulting room the question is how, by seriously taking care of her body, Henriette Tilstra can hope to be taken seriously when she speaks.

In the consulting room a body is not a precondition for the life of the mind that philosophers hold so dear. It lives, the body does, and the ideal is for it to live well. Whereas civilised citizens must tame their passions, patients in the consulting room are not asked to do so. What is wrong with passions – with lust, even? Within the logic of care, nothing. Pleasure is not low down some hierarchy or other. It is best to enjoy life while it lasts! This may sound strange, particularly in the context of diabetes care. After all: people with diabetes are encouraged to be moderate. Attending to their sugar balance often means that they need to abstain from the pleasures of the body. An occasional beer is fine, but don't make it a habit, and don't have two. One slice of cake is enough even if the party goes on. People with diabetes do not simply have to restrain themselves in meetings (like everyone else), but also in pubs, at birthday parties and in other situations where celebration takes the shape of sharing food and drink. But however hard this may be, it is not a matter of asceticism. For the crux of the modesty that care demands, is not that beer, cake and the like are bad because they give you pleasure. The point is that they will raise your blood sugar levels now, and thus prevent you from enjoying life later on. If you indulge in them at present, before long you will get complications. You will no longer be able to see, to walk. You may even die. It would be best to avoid such complications, or at least postpone them. Thus you may enjoy life a little longer. In the logic of care it makes sense to give up some pleasures if other pleasures are likely to result from this. In and of itself, pleasure is fine.

In the consulting room people with diabetes describe how difficult it is to follow the rules that come with their treatment. 'I have sinned, doctor,' they say. The occasional doctor may gravely deplore this sinning, but good professionals do not go along with such self-moralising. Instead, they calmly reply: 'Well, the reins cannot always be tight.' In the consulting room it is not a sin to enjoy yourself. It is not even looked down on. Take sex. In the diabetes outpatient clinic, conversations about sex tend to concentrate on the question how to improve a patient's 'sex life'. They are about pleasure, enjoyment, orgasms. Diabetes can be difficult in bed. There are people who occasionally get a hypo from making love (and then they may fear it will happen again). There are men with diabetes who (far earlier than they might have expected) cannot get an erection. Relationships may become difficult because one partner has the disease and the other finds the complexities that follow too difficult to handle. In such situations, good professionals talk with their patients about what might be done to improve things. Who could do what differently? How to live well? Pleasure is not a problem within diabetes care. A bad sugar balance is. Or a lack of pleasure.

Things rarely go smoothly. There tend to be frictions. Doctors and patients sometimes laugh about the irreducibilities, the things that do not fit. So you had a third beer, did you? You never went to sleep that night of the party, and you lost count of how much insulin to inject and when? That is the way it goes. These things happen. But if you really no longer care, doctors will get serious again. No, they will not say that you should be ashamed of yourself, for that leads to self-castigation, not self-care. It does not help to moralise. So instead they may say: 'Gosh, this isn't going well, is it? What is going on?' Or: 'What is troubling you?' The art of such conversations is to bring out and discuss what stops people from taking good care of themselves. The aim is to improve the situation. Yes, health care meddles with every detail of our daily lives. And indeed, it tries to normalise our bodies. But it does not despise them.[9] Care has little to do with repressing and all the more with cherishing our bodies.

Determined or alive

The 'citizen' that figures in political theory may be either Greek or civilised, and then there is a third variant as well. The citizen may also be *enlightened*. The enlightened citizen is a free spirit. A free spirit is capable of making critical judgements, insofar as he has succeeded in breaking free from worldly phenomena, including his body. Thus, he does not control his body, this citizen. Instead he escapes from it, transcends it. Like the Kantian philosopher, after whom he is modelled, the enlightened citizen disentangles himself from mere phenomena. From a reflective distance he passes normative judgements about the world. Someone who is overwhelmed by pain, is shaking with fever, fears he is dying, or whose blood sugar levels are too low, cannot, at the same time, be an enlightened citizen. Disturbing physicalities draw a person inside his body. Only when he is escaping from the flesh can an enlightened citizen become a free spirit, able to judge. Autonomously.[10]

The body of the enlightened citizen hangs together in a causal way. It is a part of nature and, since the sciences are gradually catching reality in determinist schemes, sooner or later all things physical will be explained. They form a strange pair: the free spirit celebrated by modern philosophy and the deterministic body known by modern science. But a pair they are. While political philosophy invented the enlightened citizen, natural philosophy experimented with bodily functions in the laboratory. That bodies produce gastric juice when they smell food was discovered by making dogs smell meat and then cutting their stomachs open before they had a chance to eat; or by making a small cut that allowed the gastric juice to drip out through a tube. That a pancreas produces insulin when blood sugar levels increase, was discovered by removing the pancreas from a few healthy dogs: they promptly got diabetes. And so on. The facts revealed were cast in a causal format. An increase in a body's blood sugar level causes it to produce insulin, which causes the cells to absorb sugar. A decrease in a body's blood sugar levels causes it to produce glucagon, which in turn causes the release of sugar supplies, so that blood sugar levels start to increase again. The causal chains suggest that these things are unavoidable. Whatever happens is contained in the factors that explain it.[11]

Current medicine is informed by the natural sciences. So you might think that deterministic, causal bodies would be of overwhelming relevance in the clinic. And if this were true, a plea for citizenship in the consulting room might make sense. Who, after all, wants to be reduced to an unfree body when the alternative is to be a free spirit? However, are bodies indeed addressed as causal chains in clinical settings? What if they are not? It may well be that the 'causal body' is only being introduced in the consulting room along with the ideal of citizenship. In care practices, bodies were never something one might, or should try to, escape from. They are to be cherished. And when it comes to the task of dealing with disease, a body is hardly something to which you may be reduced either. In the logic of care flesh and blood do not imply determinism. This is because, while knowledge from the natural sciences is mobilised in the consulting room, it is also given a new assignment. It is not asked to explain what the world is like, but asked to suggest what might be *done*. It is made to answer practical questions.[12]

In the consulting room the doctor asks: 'How much do you drink, Mrs Alzari?' Mrs Alzari says that she drinks four litres a day. That is a lot. However, the doctor does not understand this excessive drinking as a causal effect, but as a symptom of diabetes. And its interest is not that it reveals what happens beneath Mrs Alzari's skin, but that it points to what the doctor and Mrs Alzari might do. They would do well to act so as to find out what to do about this excessive drinking. Instead of accepting causal relations for what they are, the logic of care seeks to intervene in the lived reality of bodies. Pathophysiology may explain that a lack of insulin causes death, but in the consulting room doctor and patient are more interested in the possibilities of survival. So the doctor takes out a few forms and ticks some of the preprinted boxes. When the consultation is over, Mrs Alzari walks to the laboratory, passes urine into a jar, and gives this to a technician. She allows another technician to take blood from a vein in her arm and separate it out in various test tubes. The technician sticks labels on the jar and on the different test tubes. Then machines are put to use to measure the relevant parameters. Are they deviant? If so then more needs to be done: treatment is called for. Within the logic of care bodies are not trapped in causal chains. Rather, they are embedded in treatment practices.

In the consulting room, then, what matters is not natural laws of the body, but technical interventions in the body. Therapy is the horizon of care practices. What is more: even fact-finding itself depends on interventions. Claims about what happens inside a body always depend on something that needs to be done to the body in order to make this claim. The causal schemes of a textbook may mention 'blood sugar levels' as if they were a given, but in the consulting room nothing is ever 'given'. First, it needs to be measured. There needs to be a machine, someone to operate it, fresh blood, and someone willing to give that blood. Representations of the body as causally coherent depend on practices of examination. The textbook may hide those practices, but the consulting room cannot. An examination is something that may be done – or left undone. Is it worth the effort (the cost, the risks, what have you)? To measure or not to measure: in the consulting room this is a question that necessarily comes before the facts.

The body in the consulting room is not a causally coherent entity. It is not even a passive object of measurement and treatment practices. Instead, in the logic of care the body is active. It has to be. Unless Mrs Alzari passes urine, the laboratory technician cannot test whether her urine contains sugar. On those rare occasions that a patient refuses to be investigated, it becomes all the more apparent that most patients are putting a lot of effort into care. They wilfully collaborate with technicians and nurses. And they actively learn from them. Within a few weeks, Mrs Alzari will inject her own insulin with her own hands. And if all goes well, she will learn to prick her own fingers in order to measure her blood sugar levels. She will read the results on the display of her little monitor, so long as her eyes are good enough. Thus, the body relevant to the logic of care is not a body to which you are reduced. Taking care of yourself is (among other things) also a physical competence: it requires you to educate and train your body. When the diabetes nurse teaches Mrs Alzari how to inject her insulin – 'Yes, this is how you hold the pen. And now, yes, there, with your other hand, hold your skin. Very good.' – she does not reduce her to a body. Instead, the nurse hands Mrs Alzari the bodily skills that allow her to stay alive.[13]

In order to stay alive, a body cannot just hang together causally. It has to act. Our bodies are involved in our actions. They are even needed for making judgements. But, no, the term is not quite right. For 'making judgements' is the ability that 'free spirits' acquire by escaping from their bodies. What active patients do might better be termed 'appreciating'. Henriette Tilstra does not suspect that her blood sugar levels are low because she has freed herself from her body. On the contrary: she feels dizzy, light-headed or irritated – from the inside. One may recognise the early warning signs of upcoming hypos, not by transcending one's body but by inhabiting it. Such intro-sensing is an intriguing skill that (if your diabetes does not interfere with your senses too much) may be trained. Thus, while appreciation involves bodies, it does not happen to them. Instead it depends on the abilities and efforts of the patients who appreciate.[14] And so it is for professionals too. Long before machines are put to use clinicians diagnose with their senses. They notice posture, muscle tone and bruises; they hear sadness in a tone of voice or the signs of impaired breathing; they feel for the pulse, for lumps; and they may smell metabolic disturbances.[15] The nurse touches the spot where Mrs Alzari has been injecting her own insulin during the past week to find out whether or not the skin has hardened. The doctor shakes the hand of the next patient and finds that it is clammy. 'How are you?' We do not engage in care despite, but with, our bodies.

Who is in charge or what to do

The logic of choice is drawn into health care with the promise that it will free patients from the patriarchal rule of professionals. But professionals are not quite feudal lords. Certainly, there are situations where professionals have a lot of power, but this tends to be due to the law. The law wants professionals to decide which people are too mad to function as citizens and thus should be locked up in a closed ward. The law states that people with a contagious disease may, under some conditions, be given medication against their will. In many countries the law even asks doctors to sign papers that stipulate whether a person with diabetes is capable of driving a car or not. However, such combinations of state rule and medical control are relatively rare. More often than not, professionals in consulting rooms have a lot less power over their patients. The physician who prescribes insulin to Mrs Alzari has no way of forcing her to inject this insulin once she returns home. While people can be punished for breaking the law, failing to observe medical advice only rarely leads to sanctions.[16] It does, however, lead to other problems. If Mrs Alzari, or anyone else with type 1 diabetes, does not inject the insulin prescribed to her, she will soon feel bad and before long she will die. If she were to shoot up all the insulin in her fridge in one go, she would die even faster. Who could stop her? But patients only rarely refuse all insulin or inject a lethal dose. This is not because they are being bossed around. Instead, most people do not want to die: they would rather live. This is why they visit health-care professionals. They are ill. And even if doctors and nurses are not always as helpful as they might be, patients suffer first and foremost from their diabetes.

If you have a potentially lethal disease and there is a drug like insulin that is likely to allow you to live for quite a while longer, what do you do? When they talk about this, most patients say: 'I have no choice.' But this lack of choice does not call for emancipation. That they feel no freedom is not because they have been submitted to the force of an authority. Something else is going on. Once dead, you have no choices left at all. And life with diabetes may be tough, but it is life. It may, in many ways, be a good life too. That is what people seek. In that context their first concern is not with who is in charge, but with what to do. How to live? How to live with/in/as a body that is both fragile and able to experience pleasure? While citizens have to control, tame or transcend their bodies so as to be able to choose, patients have to find a way of nursing, fostering and enjoying theirs so as to lead a good life. All kinds of questions follow from this. What to go for, what to let go; which results are worth what kind of effort? And, most of all, what can be realised in practice? While citizenship is a way of celebrating autonomy, *patientism* is about exploring ways of shaping a good life. And then something changes and you have to start all over again. Exploring how a good life may be lived is, just like diabetes, chronic.

4   Managing versus doctoring

In the market variant of the logic of choice patients are called customers, while in the civic variant they are modelled after citizens. The first variant cannot begin to understand disease, the second wants us to control our bodies instead of nourishing them. What the two have in common is something that so far has not been made explicit. This is a specific understanding of the character of scientific knowledge, medical technologies and the tasks of professionals. Within the logic of choice scientific knowledge is taken to be a growing collection of facts that gradually increases in certainty. Professionals need to know these facts. Preferably they should also add to them. Where appropriate they should be passing them on to lay people: one of their tasks is to provide patients with information. With the relevant facts laid out, someone has to determine the value of various possible courses of action. What might be better? A pen or a pump? Tight or mild regulation? This insulin or that one? Once a decision is made, providing or implementing the chosen technique is a professional task again. But, as making the decision is a matter of balancing values, there is no particular reason why doctors or nurses should be doing this. Since treatment interferes with the life of patients, it is the values of patients that should count for most. Framed in this way, the logic seems inescapable. And it is: in the logic of choice. But not in the logic of care.

In this chapter I try to articulate how scientific knowledge and medical technology figure within the logic of care. What makes it difficult to do this, is that almost all discussions about knowledge and technology are framed in a rationalist repertoire. Most doctors,

nurses, patients and certainly most managers, researchers and policymakers would nod their heads if they were to read what I have just
written about professional practice. Yes, that is the way it works, or
should do. However, if they are probed with questions, these same
people are likely to tell stories that do not fit the rationalist picture.
Complex stories, in which facts and values intertwine. Surprising
stories, in which technologies do not live up to their promise. Stories
with strange twists and turns that are difficult to understand. Usually,
these complexities are cast as distracting disturbances. They are taken
to be signs of the messiness of mundane practices that fail to submit
to theoretical ideals. That they so fail, however, is no reason to doubt
the ideals. But is this right? Should clinicians indeed feel embarrassed
about the gap between well-ordered theories that tell them how to
handle science and technology and the far messier practices in their
consulting rooms? Is it appropriate for managers to express disdain
for what they call the 'unruliness' of doctors and nurses? Maybe not.
Maybe it is time to have a closer look at what happens in consulting
rooms and think about revising our theories about scientific knowledge, medical technology and the tasks of health-care professionals.
For all of these make quite different sense in the logic of care.[1]

Informative facts or target values

In the consulting room of the diabetes outpatient clinic a doctor and a
patient face each other. Mr Zomer has only recently been diagnosed.
He does not yet fully grasp what having diabetes is likely to involve.
Today therefore the doctor will explain a few things to him. So there
they are, ready for a difficult conversation. What is going on here: do
we witness a moment where a professional engages in the task of
'providing value-free information'? No, we don't. In circumstances
like this, or so the logic of care has it, passing a package of bare facts
across the table by talking clearly, or by handing out a coloured
brochure, is not enough. Mr Zomer is not a student who needs to
acquire knowledge about diabetes but a patient who has to learn to
live with it. Living with diabetes is going to take a lot of his time and
a great deal of his practical and emotional energy. And since it is also
likely to lead to unpleasant complications, it would be absurd to
assume that the facts that are to be explained are value-free. They are
nasty. Confronting their negative character is a requirement of good

care. You have diabetes: that is bad. At the same time, however, patients should not get overwhelmed by misery. Thus, the doctor will stress that, fortunately, there are good treatments for diabetes these days. The balance is precarious. There should be space for sadness, but not too much. A doctor should offer consolation, but also encouragement. And while suffering must be recognised as bad, the disease must simultaneously be accepted as something that needs to be dealt with in one way or another as life goes on.

The logic of care wants professionals not to treat facts as neutral information, but to attend to their values. And values come into play long before the moment when the facts have to be explained to a patient. Take the situation in which someone's blood sugar level is found to be 15 mmol/l. This is not a neutral fact, but one that is deviant: 15 mmol/l is too high. In the hospital, blood sugar levels (as well as urea concentrations, haemoglobin levels and other results of laboratory measurements) are therefore not even called facts. They are called values: blood values. Measuring blood values is an important aspect of the treatment of, and life with, diabetes. A body with diabetes is unable to regulate its own blood sugar levels from within. In bodies without diabetes, an increase in blood sugar level leads to an increase in insulin level and this insulin then instructs the cells of those bodies to absorb sugar. In diabetes this feedback system fails. After a meal blood sugar levels rise, unless you inject insulin from the outside. When you have injected insulin, blood sugar levels decrease as the cells burn up or stock the sugar they can now absorb. As blood sugar levels get lower, bodies without diabetes start to produce glucagon which releases the body's sugar supplies. In people with diabetes, this counter-regulation does not work properly. Thus the blood sugar levels of people with diabetes will get too low unless they intervene once again from the outside and eat something. Really low blood sugars make people slide into a coma. In that state they are unable to eat and need other people to inject glucagon for them.

All of this implies that blood sugar levels are fact-values. They acquire their significance from their relation to a standard: the normal blood sugar level. But this *normative fact*, the normal blood sugar level, is not a simple given either.[2] It is not something 'we' know for a fact, with solid certainty. This may sound strange. Surely something as banal as the normal value of human blood sugar levels should by now have been unambiguously established? But it has not.

The extremes are easy: a blood sugar level of 15 mmol/l is too high and one of 2 mmol/l is too low. Interestingly, these particular fact-values also leave little room for choice. A blood sugar level of 15 is so damaging that, if the body is not protected from it, it will seriously suffer. And if someone with a blood sugar level of 2 calmly considers her options, then soon she will have no options left. Come on now, eat! But where are the limits, at what point does normality stop and intervention begin?

First, let us look at the lower limit. When precisely does a blood sugar level (plasma glucose level) become too low? When, to use the medical term, does hypoglycaemia begin? The Dutch textbook *Diabetes Mellitus* reads as follows (I translate): 'For people without diabetes mellitus, blood sugar levels vary between 3 and 8 mmol/l, depending on the amount of time that has elapsed since their last meal. In general, for diabetes patients a blood glucose level of 3.5 mmol/l is used as a criterion for hypoglycaemia.'[3] The author (Timon van Haeften) does not mention it in this quotation, but if your blood sugar level falls below 3.5 mmol/l you begin to feel dizzy and irritable. Another quote. The doctoral thesis *Insulin Induced Hypoglycaemia and Glucose Counterregulation* (written by Edith ter Braak) mentions another cut-off point for hypoglycaemia: 'Hypoglycaemia may be defined as a blood glucose level of less than 3.9 mmol/l, since glucose counter-regulation in healthy people begins at this value.'[4]

These two numbers do not come from different countries or specialisms. They both come from hospital Z. Van Haeften even co-supervised the research of Ter Braak (he is gratefully mentioned in her acknowledgements). And yet these are different numbers. The implication is not that one of the numbers is true and the other an error, nor that a controversy was going on. Rather it is that numbers are adaptable. Both authors know this very well, so they avoid strong claims. They modulate their definitions with an 'in general' or a '*may be defined*'. It may be done differently as well; there are specific cases where other definitions are in order. The body does not dictate which number to use, since it does not know what the number will be used for. This depends on practice. Thus, the textbook, aimed at (future) physicians in consulting rooms, mentions a lower limit of 3.5 mmol/l. As this is the blood value where people may begin to feel their own hypoglycaemia, it is most useful in helping doctors to understand the stories of their patients. It is also good information to pass on to patients, since it fits with their own physical experiences. You may learn to realise at this point that you had better eat something. By contrast, the doctoral thesis describes research on hypoglycaemia and glucose counter-regulation. In that context 3.9 mmol/l is the more helpful lower limit to work with, because this is the blood sugar level at which (in people without diabetes) counter-regulation begins.

Within the logic of care the blood sugar level's lower limit is not a factual given that precedes decisions about what to do. But this implies that in the process of care it is not possible to put the facts on the table first, to then add the values, so as to finally decide what to do.[5] This is not to say that facts mould themselves to our wishes. Instead, the point is that practices informed by the logic of care do not proceed in a linear manner. Instead, a 'sensible course of action' and the 'normative facts' relevant to it, co-constitute each other. Care practices are resilient as well as adaptable. A good cut-off point is specific, not general. It depends on such things as the effort involved in taking a measurement; your ability to feel your hypos coming on; and whether or not you still want to work in the garden or go for a walk. It depends on the practices you are involved in. Something similar is also true for the upper limit of a normal blood sugar level. According to the textbook *Diabetes Mellitus*, 8 mmol/l is the highest value that the blood sugar levels of people without diabetes usually reach. However, this is not a very useful fact for people with diabetes. As they need to regulate their blood sugar level from the outside, the 'upper limit' they are concerned with is not so much a fact as a task. It is the blood sugar level that they have to stay below through balancing the acts of injecting, eating, exercising and so on. This blood sugar level is set for them, or they work it out jointly with their doctors, and it is called a 'target value'.

Clinical epidemiology research indicates that it is sensible to avoid having blood sugar levels of more than 10 mmol/l. Someone whose blood sugars remain below this limit most of the time runs less risk of developing the complications of diabetes (such as blindness, atherosclerosis and neuropathy). However, this does not imply that staying below 10 mmol/l is a good target value for everyone all the time. It has only become within reach at all since the introduction of fast-release insulin, which you can inject before each meal. It was imposs-

ible to achieve an upper limit of 10 mmol/l when people with diabetes injected slow-release insulin and did so only once a day. For
people who have just been diagnosed, or who are going through a
bad period in their lives, a limit of 10 mmol/l tends to be too high as
well. Just as it is for people who are overwhelmed by a sense of
failure when they have a measurement of 11 once in a while. Within
the logic of care, a good target value is one that may be achieved in
practice. One that is technologically possible and doesn't spoil
people's daily lives too much. This is the reason why a target value
cannot be passed on as a simple piece of information from the start.
Within the logic of care, identifying a suitable target value is not a
condition for, but a part of, treatment. Instead of establishing it
before you engage in action, you keep on searching for it while you
act.[6]

Means or modifiers

So the logic of choice tries to separate facts from values while the
logic of care attends to them jointly. But there is more. Another
striking difference is linked with this. The facts that the logic of
choice wants to lay out represent a disease that is located within the
patient's body. The fact-values relevant to the logic of care cannot be
laid out at all. Since they concern a disease that interferes with a
patient's life, they do not refer to a three-dimensional object (a body)
but to something historical (a life). Thus they cannot be brought
together at a single place or time. Instead, they are a part of ongoing
practices: practices of care as well as practices to do with work,
school, family, friends, holidays and everything else that might be
important in a person's life. Fact-values emerge from life just as they
interfere with it. What follows is that for the logic of care gathering
knowledge is not a matter of providing better maps *of* reality, but of
crafting more bearable ways of living *with*, or *in*, reality. True clinicians submit their interest in, say, the pancreas and the hormones
that it fails to produce, to their concern with life with a disease. Life
with a disease does not begin once all the facts have been assembled,
because gathering fact-values is an intervention in a person's life to
begin with. Prick blood. Put it in a machine. Read the results. Activities such as these are part of life with diabetes as this is shaped by
current treatment practices.

Within the logic of choice intervention begins at a later stage. Only once the values are balanced and a decision has been made, does it become possible to act – that is, to start treatment. The technologies involved in that treatment are taken to be 'means'. They serve an end. The idea is that when patients are making a choice, they decide about this end. A professional then has to come up with the best means of achieving it. The professional literature presents these means. Clinical epidemiology has developed clinical trials as research tools to inquire into the effectiveness and effectivity of treatments. Clinical epidemiology itself however, relates to patient choice in an ambivalent way. Sometimes it indeed presents its trials as tools that increase knowledge of the 'means' that doctors have at their disposal, suggesting that the 'ends' can be established elsewhere. At other times, however, clinical epidemiology casts patient choice as superfluous. For if trials show which treatments are more effective and efficient than their alternatives, there is no further need to make decisions. Just go for the treatments the trials show to be best! To the adherents of this line of thought, it is a great puzzle: why do professionals not comply? Why do they refuse to implement the results of front-line clinical trials? There is a lot going on here, but let me just note that this question fails to recognise that the parameters explored in trials, their measures of success, do not necessarily map onto the ends that patients and their doctors may want to achieve. If there are different treatments, the question is not just which of them is more effective, but also which effects are more desirable. The question is not just which treatment has the greatest impact on a given parameter, but also which parameter to measure. In chronic diseases 'health' is out of reach, so it is not obvious which parameter to go for. Different treatments may well improve different parameters. Or, to put it in the terms used in the logic of choice: not all technologies serve the same ends and not all ends are equally worthwhile to everyone concerned.

Countering a simplified belief in 'science' as the answer to all questions, the logic of choice stresses the multiplicity of medical possibilities. This makes good sense. In its turn, however, the logic of choice simplifies the relation between means and ends. It suggests that, if you choose where you want to go, your technologies will get you there. However, in the consulting room it quickly becomes clear that technologies are not obedient means: they rarely subordinate

themselves to their official ends.[7] Instead of improving a single parameter, they have an excess of, sometimes unexpected, effects. This is
the case for all kinds of interventions. Take the apparently simple,
low-tech, sugar-free diet. Before the invention of injectable insulin,
there was an experimental treatment that consisted of removing all
carbohydrates from the diets of people with diabetes. This slightly
slowed the speed with which they died. Once insulin injections
became available, such drastic diets became obsolete. However, for
decades people with diabetes were still advised to avoid sugar. This
limited their total intake of glucose and prevented the sudden blood
sugar rushes that follow from eating sugar. Both ends were beyond
dispute. But what about the means? Avoiding sugar was unpleasant.
Many people like a sweet taste. What is more, dieting singled out
people with diabetes as deviant, as different from those round about
them who enjoyed ice cream and cake. Once sugar-free variants of
sweet products appeared on the market, things became easier. But
while their sweetness was pleasant, sugar-free ice cream and cake
still set people with diabetes apart.

No wonder then, that a lot of people with diabetes were happy
when they were no longer advised to avoid all sugar. At some point,
partly because of the introduction of fast-releasing insulin that could
be injected before each meal, the treatment regimen changed. While
it remained important to try to keep blood sugar levels stable, absti-
nence was replaced with a new magic word: balance. People now
have to balance their energy intake, their insulin dose and their exercise. This means that you can have your cake and eat it, so long as
you burn up what you eat. If you go for a walk, you even have to take
something sweet with you in order to prevent possible hypos. Adap-
tive calculations have replaced relentless restrictions. But this is not
without its own unanticipated problems. In the old days, or so one of
our informants told us, when people had a birthday party, they
would buy a special sugar-free treat for you. You were an exception.
Now you can eat the same food everybody else eats. But this means
that you are also called upon to behave like everybody else. Have
some cake, people say, you did last time. You are allowed cake,
aren't you? Come, join in. It is not easy to handle moments like that,
for it is hard to refuse and say 'no'. The complicated story about carbohydrate balance appears to be more difficult to explain than the
simple story that all sugar is forbidden. The sugar-free diet made the

dividing line between 'people with diabetes' and 'people without diabetes' clearly visible. Now, because sugar-free cake no longer does
this for them, people with diabetes have to maintain this dividing line
all by themselves.

It was never one of the goals of sugar-free diets to protect people
with diabetes against the meddling of others. That it had this effect
only arose retrospectively, after the diet had changed. Technologies
always have unexpected effects: they generate forms of pain and
pleasure that nobody predicted. While for anthropologists of technology this might be a fascinating insight, in the logic of care it is something that points to a task. Good care requires that something be
done with it. Watch out for the ways in which your 'means' mess up
your 'ends'. Do not just pay attention to what technologies are supposed to do, but also to what they happen to do, even if this is unexpected. This means that good professionals need to ask patients about
their experiences and attend carefully to what they are told, even if
there is nothing about it in the clinical trial literature. There won't
be. The unexpected is not included in the design of trials. The parameters to be measured are laid out in the first stage of a clinical epidemiology research project. If doctors and nurses want to learn about
the unexpected effects of interventions, they should treat every
single intervention as yet another experiment. They should, again
and again, be attentive to whatever it is that emerges.[8]

Technologies do more than is expected of them. What is more:
they also change expectations. Take blood sugar monitors. Before
these miniaturised machines existed people's blood sugars were
measured in the laboratory once every three months or so, in the
early morning before breakfast. If the fasting blood sugar levels measured in this way were less than 10 mmol/l everyone was pleased. If
they were higher, a doctor might adjust your insulin dose the next
time you came to the outpatient clinic. Sometimes people went to
the lab a few days in a row, or came back several times on a single
day. But unless you were admitted to the hospital, that was it. Miniaturised blood sugar monitors allow for far more frequent measurements since patients can carry them around. Using a monitor, you
can measure your blood sugar levels yourself, between other daily
activities. More frequent measurement in its turn, allows for better
calibrated doses of insulin. And this has changed treatment goals.

Where it used to be good if fasting blood sugar levels remained below 10 mmol/l, now 10 mmol/l can (in many cases) be set as a target level for the whole day.[9] Thus this small machine has changed the blood values it set out to measure. Instead of behaving as a modest means, it has interfered with its own ends.

Blood sugar monitors have changed what they were meant to do, but they have not done so alone. Strict regulation, in which blood sugars are kept below 10 mmol/l all day if possible, depends on other things as well: fast-release insulin; trial results showing that strict regulation reduces complications; doctors trusting their patients' ability to look after themselves; patients willing to spend a lot of effort on self-care; daily lives in which this is possible. All of these things have jointly changed the treatment regime. But this, in its turn, has led to new problems. The incidence of hypoglycaemia has increased. If blood sugar levels are lower on average, then they are more often too low. This is not surprising, but it is annoying. Interestingly, the same blood sugar monitor that has helped to cause this problem, forms part of its solution. If you have doubts about your blood sugar level, this little machine allows you to check whether indeed you should eat something. You may feel bad because your blood sugar level has just dropped from 15 mmol/l to 8 mmol/l. If that is the case it is unwise to eat. But if your blood sugar level has just dropped to 4 mmol/l, you had better have an apple or a sandwich. So if you take the trouble to use it, your monitor warns you against eating when it would be unwise to do so even if you feel bad, while it encourages you to eat if this is needed to avoid a hypoglycaemia. Somewhere along the way, then, the blood sugar monitor has changed itself. Initially a tool for avoiding high blood sugar levels, it now also helps to prevent blood sugar levels falling too low.[10]

In the logic of choice technologies are instruments. This sounds tautological. Of course technologies are instruments. They are means to ends and the more effective these means are, the better. But what if technologies have unexpected effects? What if they go beyond, and indeed transform, the ends they are supposed to serve? Technologies are unruly. Once introduced into a world where they interfere in unexpected ways with lots of other erratic entities and configurations, they change much more than they were intended to, and are ultimately transformed themselves as well. Instead of being modest means, they are inventive mediators. The logic of care is attuned to this. It assumes that things are just as unpredictable as people. It does not take technologies to be 'mere' instruments. Instead, good care involves a persistent attempt to tame technologies that are just as persistently wild. Keep a close eye on your tools, adapt them to your needs, or adapt yourself to theirs. Technologies do not subject themselves to what we wish them to do, but interfere with who we are.

Calculating or attuning

In the logic of choice all fluidity is located in the moment choices are being made. At that moment the facts are given, and so too are the possible courses of action. But the way the various values involved will add together has yet to crystallise. What to do? This or that, A or B? That is the question. In the logic of care fluidity and solidity are distributed differently. They cannot be separated out so easily. Let us take another look at what happens in the consulting room. Sometimes this may indeed be glossed as a matter of weighing up the advantages and disadvantages of alternative options. Take the situation of Dirk Gevaert. He is 32 years old and has a small company. Not only is he the director of this company, but he also travels by car for personal visits to his clients. The last thing he wants is to get a hypo while he is driving (he does not want to have an accident, and neither does he want to be caught by the police driving badly and have his licence taken away). Thus, in order to avoid getting hypos, he takes care to eat enough and not inject too much insulin. But this isn't ideal, for in this way he keeps his blood sugar levels fairly high. Thus his risk of developing complications is high as well. If he were to set his target levels lower in order to avoid long-term trouble, this might mean that he has to give up his work. But he takes pride in his work and it provides him and the people working for him with an income. What to do? If Dirk Gevaert keeps his blood sugar levels so high that he is no danger on the road, then he is a danger to himself. But if he gives priority to his future eyesight, he loses his company. The typical clinical mode of handling such difficult questions is to seek a compromise, but sometimes a compromise is hard to craft. If so, a choice has to be made.

In the consulting room, then, doctor and patient often talk about what to value most. Or patients go home with a dilemma to think through and talk about with their 'relevant others'. But even more often, the most pressing question is not what it might be best to do, but what can be done. What can be achieved in practice? Will and desire may count for a lot, but they are rarely decisive. Take Dirk Gevaert again: if he lived in a country where he had no alternative way to earn a living, he would not have a choice either. The practicalities needing to be addressed take many forms. Let us go back to Mr Zomer. Earlier in this chapter he was told that he has diabetes. In the month that followed he gradually got used to living with this disease. He learned to inject insulin and has adapted his eating habits. Now his physician explains to him that research has shown that tight regulation reduces his chances of developing complications. 'This is something you might want to consider, Mr Zomer,' she says. She adds that tight regulation would mean that he would need to measure his own blood sugar levels regularly. If he records the results and brings them along to the next consultation, then she – the physician – will prescribe a more accurate, slightly higher, dose of insulin. He could begin by taking five measurements one working day a week. 'What do you think?' Mr Zomer looks thoughtful. And then he nods. Yes, this seems like a good idea to him. Of course he wants better eyesight, better arteries and less neuropathy in the years to come. All this sounds as if it is definitely worth the effort of measuring his blood sugar levels.

So far, this scene fits nicely within the logic of choice. A decent doctor, too: she properly provides her patient with information and leaves the decision to him. Alas, at the next visit, there are hardly any numbers in the notebook in which Mr Zomer was supposed to write down the results of his measurements. What is going on here? In the logic of choice, this situation suggests that maybe Mr Zomer does not really want to bother with tight regulation. Once he started to realise the disadvantages of all the measuring required, he may have come to another conclusion. Or maybe he has changed his mind for some other reason. Either way, if he does not want to measure then so be it. It is his own choice. In the logic of care this makes little sense. A good health-care professional will not think that Mr Zomer changed his mind once he got home, but rather that measuring turned out to be too difficult to *do*. Something that sounded fine in the consulting room turned out to be hard to carry out in daily life. These things happen. But faltering attempts are not necessarily moments of conclusion. There he is again, Mr Zomer, sitting in a chair facing his doctor. He would still like to try tight regulation if only this could be done. So care goes on. The ideal doctor begins with a comforting: 'That must have been disappointing for you, then, Mr Zomer, that it was more difficult than you thought it would be.' Moralising doesn't help. Stronger still, instilling feelings of guilt should be avoided, for these can be counter-productive. Guilty people deserve punishment, not care. How then, if you feel guilty, do you engage in self-care activities?

Thus, emotional support that facilitates self-care is a first necessary step. But it is not enough. The next task is to disentangle the practicalities Mr Zomer has to deal with when it comes to measuring his blood sugar levels. Is there something that may be slightly changed, so that next time around Mr Zomer stands a better chance of succeeding? If his measuring skills are falling short, a diabetes nurse may lead him through the procedure once again. Prick your finger; hold the test strip close to it; push blood onto the test-strip; place the strip in the monitor; read the result; and record it in your notebook. While they rehearse this, the nurse may notice that Mr Zomer has a device that does not suit him. He has trouble removing the screw top of the test strip container; or the display showing the results is too small; or the machine is too big and too cumbersome to carry around. If something like this is the case, she may lend him another monitor: would that work better? And she asks him questions. What exactly is it difficult to do? It may turn out that there is a problem with Mr Zomer's work. Yes, there is. He works on road construction. This makes it impossible for him to prick his finger five times a day. For he prefers not to prick with all his colleagues watching, but the mobile toilet, quite a walk, is the only place with any privacy, and it is dirty. What is more, if he would go there often, he would be accused of dodging work. He just cannot do it.

It is often far from easy to differentiate between what you do not want and what you cannot do. In the consulting room, patients and professionals tend not to waste too much time separating out desires and possibilities, but talk about them together. They discuss the intricacies of daily practices in their emotional as well as their technical detail. How to go about them? How to include treatment in your daily life without messing too much with other things that are important to you? Thus, for Mr Zomer the point is not to choose between 'measuring' or 'not-measuring', but to find out how to measure. How to go about it. The nurse suggests that Mr Zomer might try to take a single measurement five days a week instead of five measurements on a single day. 'Would that work?' Somehow technology, daily habits and people's skills and propensities have all to be mutually adjusted. This is crucial in the logic of care. It is important to attune everything to everything else. Nothing is taken to be entirely fixed or entirely fluid. Technologies, habits, hopes, everything in a patient's life may have to be adjusted. And so, as a patient, may you. Attending a course may teach you to feel the onset of your own hypos better (if your sensitivity is not yet undermined by the disease). Therapy may help you to lose your fear of blood. Or is it the doctor who has to change? She may be too hard or too soft, too fast or too slow. A communication expert may have the doctor look at her own consultations on a video and give her feedback. 'Look, here, this is a typical moment. You might have taken more time to listen to your patient here. Don't talk too much.'

The maximum fluidity that the logic of choice attributes to the moment of choice is not found there in the logic of care. You may want a lot, but reality does not necessarily conform. So you may choose to have low blood sugar levels, but suddenly, unexpectedly, they rise. You may decide to drive a car while tightly regulating your blood sugars, but, however hard you try to avoid them, this may lead to hypos. And even if you really want to take measurements, you may still fail to do so. Such is the viscosity of life. Habits, other people, material conditions: they do not submit to your wishes. You cannot do with them as you please. In any case, most of all you do not want to have diabetes. But you do. Thus, in the logic of care facts and technologies are more fluid than the logic of choice takes them to be, while will and wishes are more constrained. Less fluid. Control is not on offer. The world may well be adaptable and adjustable, but only up to a point. There are limits to what can be changed – but these limits are not obvious at the beginning. It is difficult to predict what may work and what will fail. Thus, the logic of care wants us to experiment carefully. Try, be attentive to what happens, adapt this, that or the other, and try again.[11]

In the logic of choice a good decision depends on properly balancing the advantages and disadvantages of various courses of action. The model of 'balance' mobilised here comes from accountancy. There, a financial balance has a credit and debit side. Although the advantages and disadvantages of medical interventions are more difficult to quantify than sums of money, the model is used in a strikingly similar way. It is as if making a decision were like making a calculation. Pros and cons, one side versus the other. In the logic of care this is different. 'Balance' is important once again, but not as a matter of adding and subtracting advantages and disadvantages. After all, addition and subtraction require fixed variables, but in the logic of care no variable is ever fixed. All variables are variable – to some extent. The 'balance' sought, then, is something that needs to be established, actively, by attuning viscous variables to each other. Rather than the balance sheet of the accountant, the balancing body of a high-wire artiste or a dancer come to mind. And even if finally everything fits, if everything is nicely attuned to everything else, it may all fall apart again. Your fingers lose their sensitivity. Your eyesight deteriorates. You have to care for your aging parents. Your relationship falls apart. You are made redundant at work. You want to take a long-haul flight across several time zones: how do you manage that? The logic of choice suggests that choosing is confined to specific moments. Privileged moments, difficult maybe, but bounded. The logic of care, by contrast, suggests that attuning the many viscous variables of a life to each other is a continuing process. It goes on and on, until the day you die.

Managing doctors or shared doctoring

In the logic of choice time is linear. The key moment, the moment a choice is being made, is embedded in a sequence: (neutral) facts → (value-laden) choice → (technical) action. Once the action is over, it becomes possible to evaluate it. As an afterthought. In the logic of care this is different: time twists and turns. There is no single, crucial moment when all relevant fact-values are available. Problems emerge and as they are tackled new problems arise. Fixing the target of a treatment before the treatment begins just cannot be done: establishing a target is a part of treatment. And when something unexpected turns up, it has to be integrated with everything else. Thus, in the logic of care it makes no sense to put arrows between events and order them in a linear manner. Take self-measurement: is this one of the conditions for the introduction of tight regulation, or one of its consequences? And why would one want to postpone evaluation until after the action has taken place? It makes more sense to start evaluating early on, as a part of the attempt to fine-tune treatment and improve it. In living with diabetes time is not a moment-by-moment affair. For while the past has left ineradicable traces within you, the future is already present too. You try to juggle with the future. The tight regulation in which you engage does not make you feel better now. Instead, you hope it will postpone the complications of your diabetes. It is good for later. The logic of care does not unfold in time. It folds time.

In the linear time of the logic of choice there is a marked difference between what is given and what is open for discussion. Knowledge and technologies are given. They may change over the years, but they are fixed in the brief moment that matters: the moment a choice is being made here and now. Knowledge and technology make choices possible in the first place. But they fall outside the scope of discussion. You cannot choose for or against their existence: they are given, they frame the options that are available and thus they frame the discussion. What information might be worth gathering, or which technologies worth building is not a matter of choice for individual patients in the consulting room. This has been decided earlier and somewhere else. Which methods have been used to create knowledge? Which research questions have been addressed? Which technologies have been made? And why these and not others? None of this is relevant. All the emphasis is on the choice to be made here and now. The question as to how we have ended up here and now, in this particular situation rather than in another, is not appropriate. Making a choice given this situation is difficult enough as it is.

Maybe it is so difficult that it is not surprising that many patients want professionals to make their choices for them. 'What do you think, doctor?' they say. 'What would you do if it was you; what would you advise if it was your father, mother, partner, child?' According to the logic of choice, answering such questions may sometimes be kind but it is not a professional task. Professionals should provide good information, and properly implement the interventions for which their patients opt. They should be knowledgeable, accurate and skilful. They should be capable of handling large quantities of information and able to act competently, but it is the patients who determine the direction to be taken. Patients manage, doctors implement. This is different in the logic of care. Here it is impossible to separate management and implementation. Attuning variables to each other is as much about establishing facts as it is about figuring out what to do. Using technologies requires that they be adjusted to each specific situation. Care is not a matter of implementing knowledge and technology, but of experimenting with them. To talk about the work involved, I would like to rehabilitate a word that has acquired pejorative connotations. I want to talk of *doctoring*. Within the logic of care engaging in care is a matter of doctoring. Doctoring again depends on being knowledgeable, accurate and skilful. But, added to that, it also involves being attentive, inventive, persistent and forgiving.

Doctoring is not something that only doctors do. The entire care team is involved in it. Take the case of Mr Zomer again. The doctor mentions the possibility of tight regulation. The diabetes nurse suggests that Mr Zomer collects his measurement results over five days rather than one. To allow for this she changes a page in his preprinted little notebook, so that he can note the results in a way that is still easy to read. Mr Zomer himself tries to measure his blood sugar levels, and, if he does not succeed, he goes back to the consulting room to talk things over. The crucial question in relation to doctoring is not who is in charge, but whether or not the various activities involved are well attuned to one another. Does everything and everyone cooperate or are there tensions and clashes? Maybe the nurse should take more time to listen, thus she might learn more about the difficulties her patients face in their daily lives. Attending to her patients' experiences would allow a doctor to fine-tune her own activities better. There is always something to improve. Even idealised practice is not ideal. It is a matter of trying things out and of being willing to revisit what has been done before. There is always something that fails. Try again, adjust, improve. Or, when the time is right, let go.

A team that shares the task of doctoring offers an interesting model for the democratisation of expertise. Up until now the democratisation of expertise has mostly been presented as a matter of making the demos, the people, in one form or another, rule over experts. As if from the outside. From above.[12] First, democratically governed states were called upon to control professionals. Now, in the logic of choice, patients are invited to do so individually. They must push professionals back into their cage, the place where they know the facts and handle the instruments. At the same time patients themselves are to make the crucial decisions, those that involve values. Thus, in the logic of choice patients are called upon to manage their doctors. The logic of care suggests a different way of opening up the monopoly of professional groups over expertise. Let us, somehow, share the doctoring. Let us experiment, experience and tinker together – practically. This is far from easy. Shared doctoring requires that everyone concerned should take each other's contributions seriously and at the same time attune to what bodies, machines, foodstuff and other relevant entities are doing. Those who share doctoring must respect each other's experiences, while engaging in inventive, careful experiments. They must attune all variable variables to each other, while attending to everyone's strengths and limitations. They must change whatever it takes, including themselves. Shared doctoring requires us to take nothing for granted or as given, but to seek what can be done to improve the way in which we live with our diseases. And remember that failure is inevitable and death the only security we have.

5   Individual and collective

So far this book has talked of individual patients and the ways in which 'choice' and 'care' configure their situation. However, people do not live alone, they form collectives. This chapter considers how the 'individual' and the 'collective' relate in the context of health care. Is a collective the sum total of a number of individuals added together, or can we only understand what individuals are if we first learn about the – various – collectives to which they belong? And should public health be improved by asking individuals to change their behaviour, or by interfering with the conditions in which collectives live? The logic of choice and the logic of care answer these questions in different ways. To show this, I will again talk about life with diabetes in the Netherlands. But improving 'public health' includes trying to prevent disease and currently nobody knows how to prevent type 1 diabetes. For this reason I will widen the scope of my discussion and more directly include type 2 diabetes and attempts to prevent it.

The logic of choice assumes that we start out as separate individuals and that we begin to form a collective as we are added together. This means that it frames individuals as building blocks that jointly make a larger whole. The building blocks are named in different ways. In the market variant of the logic of choice they are called 'customers'. Each customer has individual demands and in the market these are added to create an overall demand. In the civic variant of the logic of choice that informs liberal democratic societies, the individual building blocks that make up the collective are called 'citizens'. Citizens may exert influence by voting. Their votes are added together and the majority wins. Neither of these systems of addition is completely linear. For instance, in the market minority demands may be too small to count: meeting them may not be profitable. In liberal democracies small minorities of citizens sometimes count for more than their numbers. People who are outnumbered are not necessarily sidelined: good government takes 'minority interests' into account. But even if the addition is not entirely linear, in both cases collectives are a consequence of adding individuals together.

In the context of health, addition may also be used to move from individuals to the collective. This happens in liberal, individualised public health efforts. Here, collectives are not created by adding demands or votes, but by aggregating parameters. In order to do this epidemiological research and the tools of statistics are deployed. Bodily indicators of health and disease (the parameters) are measured and correlated with (a few of) the activities in which people engage. In this way particular activities are correlated with particular indicators of health or disease. Then everyone is encouraged to engage in activities that appear to bring health and to abstain from whatever correlates with disease. We are told, for instance, that we should eat in moderation (including fruit and vegetables!) and that we should take enough exercise (engage in sport, go cycling, swimming or walking). The hope is that if all individuals were to adapt their lifestyles in accordance with the ideals uncovered by research, the health of the collective would improve. In the name of public health, we are called upon to 'choose a healthy lifestyle'.

Note that in this context the character of 'choice' has changed. In previous chapters 'choice' figured as an ideal. It was said that patients *should* be allowed to make their own choices and that professionals *ought* to leave value-laden decisions to their patients. The terms used, 'should' and 'ought', suggested that things do not always work in this way. 'Choice' was framed as a normative project: granting patients the possibility of choosing is a good thing that should be put into practice. However, when public health campaigns encourage us to 'choose a healthy lifestyle', something different is happening. Suddenly it is assumed that, as it is, the way we live already follows from the choices that we make. Nobody stops you from living in a healthy way, now, do they? From an ideal that might be realised if a lot of effort were put into it, choice is suddenly turned into a fact of life. Making choices is what people do. The surprising thing is that they make such strange and unwise choices. Why do so many people choose to eat so much and exercise so little? There are even people who choose to smoke. Public health campaigns encourage us to make better choices. For if each of us, individually, opts to do the right thing, we might, added together, form a healthy collective.

In this chapter I try to show that in the logic of care none of this makes much sense. This is because the logic of care does not start with individuals but with collectives. A variety of them. Patients who present themselves in the consulting room are members of families, have colleagues, live in a street, and so on. It may be hard work to disentangle people from their collectives sufficiently for the care that they individually need. At the same time, there are collectives to which we belong that frame the care we receive, or the care that might be good for us. Diagnostic groups, genetic relatives, people with whom you share habits, a past, food – any of these may be important. But which of them actually is? The character of the collectives that are relevant to care is not given but somehow needs to be established. In this context epidemiological research is mobilised again, but in a different way. Which collectives should be categorised together? And as the conditions under which various collectives live are then correlated with the extent to which they are plagued by disease, the quest is for care that, rather than moralising individual behaviour, improves life for the collective.

The difference is profound. In the logic of choice pre-given individuals are added together to form collectives, while division may be used to move back from what counts for a collective to whatever is pertinent to the individuals who compose it. Individual and collective are set up in a transitive relation. In the logic of care, by contrast, variously categorised collectives may be separated out into individuals in various ways. The move from collectives to individuals is one of specification, while collectives, in their turn, do not result from adding individuals together, but from making helpful differentiations between groups. None of this is easy to grasp. In the pages that follow I try to outline it step by step. What are 'collective' and 'individual' made to be in health-care practices? To answer this question, I will, once again, tell you some stories.

Pre-given individuals or careful individuation

A photo of a patient and a doctor in a consulting room may seem to show two individuals meeting. There they are, sitting on opposite sides of a desk. The logic of choice would lead one to ask whether the doctor is paternalistic or whether the patient gets to choose, while presuming that there are just two people present. However, if you sit on a stool in a corner of the consulting room and listen to what is being said, you find that something else is going on. The two people visible do not act alone. Many others are linked to them. Hidden behind the doctor is the secretary who arranged the appointment; colleagues who might offer advice or make .critical comments; teachers and conference speakers; the diabetes nurse further down the hallway who is holding a visiting hour at the same time (a 'diabetes meeting' is scheduled for later in the day). In the context of this chapter, however, I am not primarily concerned with the doctor. What about the patient's hidden company? At some point, the doctor may ask: 'Is there any diabetes in your family?' With this question the patient's family enters the scene. Not the in-laws, however. The question is only about blood relatives, with whom the patient shares a gene pool. Each individual, or so genetics tells us, inherits a unique set of genes, but the pool is there first. It precedes the individual.[1] This is common knowledge: patients also often spontaneously mention previous carriers of their physical characteristics. 'Don't worry about the high blood pressure, doctor. My father had it as well, it was impossible to get it down.' For the modern doctor, a patient's 'inherited burden' is no reason to sit back and relax, but a challenge. Can a new drug be found that works where earlier ones did not? Maybe, maybe not. Either way, the high blood pressure turns the absent father into an inconvenient presence.

That patients are part of families helps in diagnosis. If diabetes genes made an earlier appearance within someone's family, then this increases the probability that they, too, have this disease. Families are also relevant for therapy. This time the in-laws are included because, instead of shared genes, now it is shared habits that are important. However, family habits do not always help in the treatment of diabetes. They may stand in its way. Take the situation of Lies Henstra, who has type 2 diabetes. Her general practitioner has been encouraging her to lose weight for some time. But in an interview she says: 'I have followed a lot of diets. I find it so difficult. Once, I lost forty kilos, but I quickly put them back on again. I could eat less, but I can't. In our family, we're food lovers. I am, I have been ever since I was a child. I just keep eating.' Family habits exist before you appear on the scene; like genes they precede you. They make you who you are. And so do the traditions of other collectives to which you belong. Tjeerd van Eerden is a salesman. 'No, it is impossible, really,' he says, 'to follow a diet. In my work, I have to take clients to a restaurant. I can't just skip a course.' It is difficult to act strangely; difficult to do something that does not fit with the company you keep. Yet this is exactly what the logic of care wants you to do. In order to take care of yourself, you may need to deviate. Dessert is served and you should say: 'No, no thank you, not for me.'

Disentangling yourself from a collective is not a question of becoming the individual you are. It has nothing to do with making space for your true self.[2] After all, if you come from a family of food lovers, then you truly are a food lover, deep down. You have been so ever since you were a child. And if your dining-room table is also your meeting-room table, you may well be a wonderful host, all the way through. The point is that you must learn to become someone different. Such 'individuation' is not easy. Let go of what is familiar. Be different. But how? One of the complications is that being marked out as deviant can be uncomfortable. As Ruud Stevens puts it in an interview: 'Early on, one of my friends was getting married. I had just left hospital. At the time I was used to having a cooked meal for lunch, and some bread in the evening. When I mentioned this to my friend, he says: no problem. We'll make sure you get bread. Don't worry. And while we are sitting there, this waiter comes into the room with my plate of bread and calls out: "Where's the diabetes patient?" Everyone could see it was me. So after that I said: never again. I'll just join in.' Joining in is nicer than being publicly marked as deviant. Luckily there are some practical formats that make it possible to combine similarities and differences. As Mrs Zirsto explains, buffets are a lot easier than dinners. With a buffet you can take the right amount of what it would be wise to eat. Nobody notices that you are doing anything special. Mrs Zirsto: 'I was very happy about that, about having a buffet at my son's wedding. It started late, though, so an hour earlier I asked for a sandwich.'

What can be differentiated and what is tied together depend on the technical details of daily life. This means that the individuation called for by the logic of care is a material as well as an emotional task. Take the family meal. Mr Regters in an interview: 'They think, lay people, that sugar is worse for your body than other things. But it's not. For me, fat is far worse. It is. So I take skimmed milk in my coffee. And I use a different type of butter. And so does my wife.' At this point his wife interrupts him rather sharply: 'Oh no, I don't. I don't like it at all.' Mr Règters continues in an appeasing manner: 'No, I don't mean on your bread. I mean for frying, that other type of butter.' One of the traditions of the Dutch cold meal (eaten twice daily) is that, if you eat it at home, slices of bread are served in a bread basket. You sit at the table together, but everyone butters their own bread (and then they put something like cheese on it, or chocolate sprinkles). While Mr Regters uses low-fat poly-unsaturated margarine to protect his arteries, Mrs Regters smears her bread with full-cream butter, because that is what she likes. But when it comes to preparing the single hot meal of the day, it is a lot easier to fry the meat in a single frying pan, all in one go. Mrs Regters cooks. And she is generous: she uses the 'other butter', the diet one that is good for her husband, for frying meat. She does not make him eat something that is bad for his arteries and neither does she isolate him as deviant. Instead, she adapts herself.

Together or apart, or a bit of both – you do what you can. But there are also collectives from which people do not want to be separated. Take Mrs Sanders: her husband has dementia and he is getting worse every day. He swears at her and sometimes he hits her as well, which he never used to do. Mrs Sanders is glad when she has to go to the hospital to get her diabetes checked, for then a home-care nurse comes to the house to take care of her husband. It gives her a break. And yet Mrs Sanders is determined to keep her husband at home for as long as she possibly can. He is in such a bad state by now that it would not be too difficult to have him admitted to the geriatric department of a nursing home. His anger is often overwhelming; Mrs Sanders has bruises; she rarely gets a good night's sleep; and she cannot attend her physical exercise class twice a week (something the doctor recommended that she should do). But, she says: 'After all we have been through together, I cannot just desert the man.' Although Mrs Sanders is perfectly capable of pointing out how difficult the bonds of marriage have become, and how bad they are for her and for her health, she does not want to disentangle herself. It would feel like a betrayal.

The logic of choice assumes that we are autonomous individuals. The logic of care is attuned to people who are first and foremost related. While some of these relations cannot be changed, others can. But even if people in part disentangle themselves from family members, friends and colleagues in order to take care of their body with diabetes, they never cut all their ties. And new entanglements develop too. These may be entanglements with other people with diabetes, whether you have met them or not. As one informant explained: 'When I see a war on tv, or refugees, these days I wonder, how about the insulin for those with diabetes? Where do they get that, how do they keep it cold?' And there are entanglements, too, with the other members of the care team. At the moment a patient refuses dessert – 'No, no thank you, not for me' – he may feel the support of his dietician or diabetes nurse – 'Very good!' And while Mrs Regters quarrels with her husband during the interview, she cooks his meat in the fat that he needs. Some of us go for a walk with a friend who says after a while: 'Shouldn't you eat something?' Nobody acts all alone. Who bakes your bread? Who removes your rubbish bags? Who writes your newspaper? The logic of choice is concerned with individuals who wish to be free. The individuals who figure in the logic of care would die if they were left alone. They owe their very ability to act to others.[3]

Adding equals or crafting categories

Individuals belong to collectives. But who forms a collective with whom? In the logic of choice we belong with others who are similar. On the market every customer is as much a customer as any other. In civic affairs all citizens should be treated in the same way. The people addressed by individualised public health campaigns are also made to be equal: they all have a 'lifestyle' and may opt for one that is better. In the logic of choice we may be unique in *what* we choose; but *that* we choose is something we share. This is celebrated as a good, as a victory over earlier, hierarchical systems in which masters were placed above servants; in which 'difference' implied hierarchy. In the logic of care we are not equal. But the difference between us has little to do with hierarchy. It does not imply that some people (professionals) are allowed to treat others (patients) as their subordinates. What matters in the logic of care are horizontal differences between people. These index different needs, and more particularly different needs for care. But how are the care-relevant differences between people framed?

In this book I talk about 'people with diabetes'. Is this a good term? Is it a sensible way of grouping people together? In the logic of care there is no general answer to a question like this. It depends on the context. The diabetes nurses whose work I observed care for a wide variety of 'people with diabetes'. Since the nursing care that 'people with diabetes' need is geared to their task of balancing their blood sugar levels from the outside, this way of framing a specialisation makes sense. But in other contexts the same clustering does not work so well. When it comes to shaping prevention practices, a distinction between 'type 1' and 'type 2' diabetes is made, because nobody knows how to prevent type 1 diabetes, whereas for type 2 diabetes there are various suggestions. In yet other contexts, it makes sense not to split the category of 'people with diabetes', but to cluster it together with other (diagnostic) groups. For example, it is sensible for everyone 'with a deviant sugar metabolism' (not only people with diabetes, but also those who have reactive hypos following sugar intake) to avoid Coca-Cola (which increases blood sugar levels too rapidly). And then there are situations like those of the physiotherapist who offers walking therapy. She may offer her care to all 'people with bad leg arteries' (irrespective of whether they are due to diabetes or not). But she may also drop disease categories altogether. In the logic of care the best strategy might well be to welcome to a walking group 'people who would do well to walk more'. For the people addressed in this way share a need to walk, whatever their diagnosis.

In the logic of care categorising is not like collecting. It is not a question of aggregating individuals with characteristics that are already there. Instead, categorising is a matter of differentiating between collectives. In the process some individual characteristics come to be framed as relevant. The category and the individual that belongs to it, are shaped together. But while categories inevitably inform identities, they may do so in different ways. In the past 'people with diabetes' were called 'diabetics'. Patient activists objected to this term, since it suggests that a person may *be* 'a diabetic'. Thus, the person's identity seems to coincide with her diagnosis. As an alternative, the term 'people with diabetes' was proposed. While being 'with diabetes', 'people with diabetes' may also play the piano, come from Amsterdam, have an Italian grandmother, like to walk, or love food. The list of attributes (and thus the relevant categories in which one might fit) is left open. In most writing (including professional papers) the new term has replaced the old. This is in accordance with the logic of care, where categories are not taken to be fixed reflections of a given reality, but tools to work with. If they don't work out well in practice, look for others. If tying a person's identity too tightly to a diagnostic category is not helpful, then look for looser kinds of links.

Some categorisations serve care practices better than others. Which categorisations might be helpful when it comes to designing prevention practices? Currently the worldwide incidence type 2 diabetes is rapidly rising. However, there are remarkable differences between populations. But between which 'populations' exactly? How do we differentiate one from the other, and categorise the people involved? In Canada it was found at one point that the incidence of type 2 diabetes was very high among the indigenous people of the country, the Inuit. This only became apparent because 'the Inuit' had already been clustered together as a 'population' in other contexts. Their ancestors hunted for fish and seals long before the 'whites' came, saw and conquered. Currently the Inuit (mostly) live grouped together in reservations, and share old traditions, recent claims on the Canadian government, and some physical features. But what might they have in common that correlates with getting type 2 diabetes? And are there any other groups that might share this characteristic?[4] In the Netherlands, for example, type 2 diabetes has a comparatively high incidence among Hindu immigrants from Surinam. In which respects do they resemble the Canadian Inuit?

Various answers circulate. A first one is: genes. The populations concerned have lived for centuries in situations where food was scarce. As a result, there has been no selection against genes that correlate with type 2 diabetes: no-one ever died of this disease, and certainly not before having children. Now that enough food is available, these genes come to expression. Framed in this way, a 'population' is a group of people who enter into endogamous marriages: they have children together and thus come to share a gene pool. 'Diabetes genes' might then characterise the 'Inuit' as well as 'Hindus'. A second answer to what 'Inuit in Canada' and 'Hindus in the Netherlands' may have in common is: habits. This is the story: people who live in conditions of scarcity begin to eat a lot if food suddenly becomes available. In the past, feasts would alternate with periods of famine, and everybody who over-ate would lose weight again. But, if there are no more periods of famine, these same people put on too much weight and, as a result, their chances of developing type 2 diabetes increase. A socio-historical concept of 'population' is at play here: a 'population' is a group that shares habits. Then there is a third answer to what the 'Inuit in Canada' and 'Hindus in the Netherlands' might share, an answer from biochemistry. A body that is malnourished early on in its development, adjusts its biochemistry to low food intake. Every calorie available is either used or stored. This biochemical specificity cannot be reversed later in life, even if by then there is plenty of food. People who were malnourished when young will put on weight even if they eat only modestly. This increases their chances of getting diabetes. This third type of 'population' gathers together people who were malnourished in the womb and as small babies. These are people who have (a part of) their life history in common.[5]

These three ways of categorising and framing 'populations' give three different glosses on what 'Canadian Inuit' or 'Hindus living in the Netherlands' might be. People who share genes; people who share habits; or people who share a personal history of malnutrition. But categorisations like these are not fixed. Suppose that further research were to reveal that the high incidence of type 2 diabetes among people who are now called 'Inuit' or 'Hindu' is indeed related to their genetic make-up. In the first instance this would reinforce a genetic understanding of populations as 'people who share genes'. This does not quite turn such populations into races, but even so this population concept has racial overtones. Races, too, were defined as populations sharing genes.[6] However, if suitable genetic tests were subsequently to become available, the genetic understanding of 'Inuit' and 'Hindu' might well dissolve again. For such tests would differentiate between people with and people without genes that make them prone to acquiring diabetes. Thus, the availability of an appropriate test might mean that only two genetic populations would end up being relevant to diabetes prevention: the population of 'carriers' and that of the 'non-carriers' of type 2 diabetes genes. In this way, more genetics might lead to a less racial understanding of who belongs with whom. Instead, disease-gene-related population categories might come to dominate.[7]

However, it also might turn out that genetics fails to explain why Inuit in Canada and Hindus in the Netherlands have more type 2 diabetes than those living around them. Maybe research will suggest habits to have the strongest explanatory power. If so, then we may expect another shift in categories. For marginalised Inuit and migrant Hindus are not the only groups with habits that follow from a history of fasting and feasting. This also goes for many other poor and formerly poor people in the world. The current character of their material surroundings makes things worse. For as it is, fat and sugar are a lot cheaper than the healthier foods most poor people have eaten in the past. Hence the worldwide increase in obesity, and, probably following on from this, a similar increase of type 2 diabetes. But if interference in food patterns is tried out as a way to prevent a further increase, identifying populations as 'Inuit' or 'Hindu' is no longer very useful. Preventive measures might rather serve 'everyone who shares a cultural history of fasting and feasting'. Or they might be aimed at 'all people who are poor but have easy access to cheap sugar and fat'.[8]

In the logic of care categories are adaptable. They have to be adapted to the tasks at hand. However, the possibility of creating and dissolving categories is not limitless. Established practices tend to be resilient. For example, almost all medical registration systems make a distinction between two sexes. Thus it is so easy to use the categories 'men' and 'women' that they get used endlessly. In this way, the distinction between the populations of 'men' and 'women' acquires ever-increasing thickness and significance. It is reinforced. This happens at the expense of other possible categorisations. In some contexts, it might be more helpful to distinguish 'people who menstruate' (who also happen to be women) and 'people who do not menstruate' (a category that not only includes men but also young girls, women after menopause and various other non-menstruating women). In other contexts (for instance when the issue is how long a drug is retained in the body) it might make sense to differentiate between 'people who have a substantial layer of subcutaneous fat' and 'people who do not'. But at present it does not work this way. Nor is it likely that the categories 'Inuit' and 'Hindu' will disappear overnight, no matter how prevention practices for type 2 diabetes are shaped and changed. Such categories are too well established in other practices. This said, the logic of care suggests that good care should not give way to other practices too easily. Instead, it should be proudly care-specific. The example is set by a group of researchers who demonstrated the biochemical irreversibility of early malnutrition. They gathered data from a group of people who had recently immigrated to Los Angeles from a very poor region of Guatemala and compared these with the (well-recorded) data about Dutch people born in the food-scarce 'starvation winter' in the Netherlands of 1944–1945. For whatever the differences between these groups, so far as their biochemical early history was concerned, they were members of the same population.

In the logic of care categories are linguistic tools that have to be fine-tuned to the task at hand. Meanwhile, the task at hand does not precede the relevant categories. A category and the practices in which it is used shape each other in a process of mutual adaptation. Back and forth it goes: terms set tasks, tasks change terms. Along the way our identities vary too. They may be made one-dimensional ('diabetics') or layered ('people with diabetes'). They may be disease-specific ('type 2 diabetes'), symptom-specific ('someone who suffers from hypos'), or action-focused ('someone who would do well to walk more'). They may confirm an identity that comes from somewhere else ('Hindu') or craft an identity that had not previously been named ('people with a tradition of feasts and famine'). The possibilities are dazzling. But the bottom line is that the question as to which categorisation is better than its alternatives does not precede care practices. It is a part of them. In the logic of care, the crucial question to ask about a category is whether or not it takes good care of you.

Healthy behaviour or helpful conditions

Individuals may be more or less healthy and so, too, may populations. How do their respective levels of health relate? If the logic of choice tries to further public health by encouraging individuals to 'choose a healthy lifestyle', then it seems to suggest that the health of the collective and that of the individuals out of which it is composed, run parallel, that they grow together. If a population is indeed the sum total of individuals added together, then this makes sense. For then the health of a population increases in proportion to the health of the individuals composing it, while individuals in their turn enjoy their fair share of the population's health. What is good for the individuals is good for the population and vice versa. It sounds self-evident: surely this must be the case? But no. If one looks in more detail at practices of care, what seems to be self-evident starts to crumble. The point is this. In the logic of care the crucial moves to make are not addition and division, but differentiation and specification.

Within the logic of care, trying to improve public health by persuading individuals to 'choose a healthy lifestyle' is not such a good idea. For a start, public health campaigns are too general, they make no differentiations. They do not distinguish between specific people and their specific situations, but address us as if we were all equal. Consider, for instance, propaganda for exercise illustrated by an image of a running figure. For a while, in order to avoid appealing to young white men only, the Dutch version of this figure had no visible age, ethnicity or gender. Recently the outline of a young woman with long, windblown hair has come to stand in for all of us. But if you happen to move around in a wheelchair then you do not see yourself reflected in running figures of any kind. And while some people with diabetes can run without getting hypos, others cannot. General appeals just remind them that they are deviant. Indeed, in one way or another, many people are. If I were to run, my knees would quickly start to hurt. If we were to talk about it, a physiotherapist would advise me to go walking rather than running. But public health campaigns do not include physiotherapists or other caring professionals who might translate generalities into the specificities suitable for particular people. While addressing us as if we were equal, they do not provide care. Good care depends on specification.

As it is, however, even differentiating the general population into sub-populations is often thought to be too complicated. Thus in the Netherlands (as in many other places), for a long time we were all encouraged to reduce our intake of cholesterol. It was claimed that this would be good for our arteries. However, even then clinical trials showed something different. Low cholesterol levels are not good for everyone: they make no positive difference for premenopausal women. Thus the general advice does not apply to the population of 'people who menstruate'.[9] But 'people who menstruate' were supposed to prepare the family meal. It was assumed that they lived with and cooked for a male partner and that he might benefit from unsaturated fatty acids. In the Netherlands there was explicit discussion about this when the guidelines were written. The conclusion was that things should not be made over-complicated.

Thus, in the hope that those who might benefit would eat less cholesterol, restricting its intake was celebrated as a general good. Nobody
told 'people who menstruate' that for them (so long as they were not
overweight) eating cheese or butter is fine. It may well be that this
message is indeed too complex to get across in a public health cam-
paign. So much the worse for campaigns. In the logic of care this way
of glossing over specificities is questionable, if only because once
people find out that the advice that they have been given does
not apply to them, they may ignore all further advice even if it is
appropriate.

Seen from the logic of care, then, the first problem with public
health campaigns is that they treat us as if we are equal, as if one size
fits all. They address people without being specific, while good care
depends on specification. There is a second problem too. A disease
that plagues a collective is not quite the same as the sum total of the
individual cases of this disease. This becomes most obvious when we
look at epidemics. For most infectious diseases, adding up the individual victims is no indication of the extent to which the infection
will hit the collective. Microbes, after all, multiply inside us. Each
sick person may infect many others and each healthy person's risk of
disease increases with the number of people infected. Thus epidemics
do not grow in a linear manner. The curves are exponential. (Until
the number of susceptible individuals gets too low.) The implication
is that microbes and liberalism do not go well together. While in liberalism every body counts for one, microbes make far wilder calculations. Thus in the nineteenth century, when larger numbers of
people started living closely together, state and city governments
learned that it was not enough to let everyone individually attend to
their own health. Someone had to intervene at a collective level.
Without serious public health efforts the microbes would have
won.[10]

Good care aimed at collectives tinkers with the conditions in
which these collectives live. The nineteenth-century public health
efforts that succeeded in making cities easier to survive in did not
take the form of pamphlets admonishing individuals to lead more
hygienic lives. Sewers and drains were built; the supply of food was
submitted to rules of hygiene; and health inspectors were
appointed. In an analogous way, the logic of care offers suggestions
for collective measures that might help to prevent diseases such as

type 2 diabetes. For even if these are not contagious, neither do they hit individuals in a random way. They may be linked to genes shared within gene pools; and they are intertwined with the collective practices that help to shape our lives. The latter are easiest to intervene in. Thus it makes sense to provide free swimming classes for specific, well-targeted groups; easily accessible swimming pools; outdoor recreational˙ areas; separate bicycle paths; more generous subsidies for sports clubs; facilities for exercise during lunch breaks; accessible paths for walking; rights of way; cooking courses; stricter food legislation (not only aimed at preventing infections and poisoning, but also at restricting people's intake of sugar and fat); interventions in food prices; suitable kinds of agriculture; and so on. Rather than telling individuals what to choose, such caring interventions would try to improve the collectively shaped conditions under which we live. Instead of obliging us to exercise our will power, they would help us to take care of our bodies.

Public health campaigns that call upon individuals to make proper choices are too general and do not take notice of the collective preconditions for individual health and disease. There is yet a third reason why what is good for the health of individuals is not necessarily good for the health of populations and vice versa. This has to do with the accounting involved. Take the example of exercise again. Running can be thrilling; walking is wonderful. A lot of people say that exercise makes them feel better. But what about the claim that it is 'healthy'? Such claims are based on measuring the effects of 'exercise' (defined in one way or another) on a few parameters (that stand in for 'health') in a population. But if positive effects are measured in this way, then we need to divide them by quite large figures to work out what they mean for you and me individually. A (simplified) example. Take a population in which 100 people out of 10,000 die of a heart attack every year. Say that research shows that, if they all start to go for a daily run, the incidence of fatal heart attacks decreases from 100 to 70. That leads to an impressive improvement: the 'health of the population' increases by 30 per cent. But what about the individuals in that population? If they start running, their probability of *not* dying from a heart attack in the course of the next year increases from 99 per cent to 99.3 per cent. This sounds much less impressive. While a decrease in deaths from heart attacks of 30 per cent is good for the population as a whole, for an individual a 0.3 per cent extra chance of avoiding a fatal heart attack (on top of the 99 per cent chance of not getting one in the first place) is a lot less appealing.

Thus, what is good for a population need not be equally good for its individual members. And this is also true the other way around. Care given to the individuals who most need it rarely improves public health. Take diabetes. People with type 1 diabetes would die without insulin, so if all care for them were stopped overnight, this might have a measurable effect on the health of the population as a whole. And if no treatment had been available, the sudden introduction of insulin would also influence population statistics. But as things stand, in Western countries relatively few people die from diabetes at an early age. It happens, but it is rare. And this is the situation from which epidemiological measurements start out when new interventions are assessed. Thus, if tomorrow some treatment were introduced that prolonged the lives of people with type 1 diabetes by, say, an average of six months, this would have no influence on the overall mortality statistics of Western countries. As the incidence of type 1 diabetes is not huge, the difference would be too small for the numbers to be significant. Improvements in care that do not prolong life, but 'only' increase the quality of life, affect public health even less. It is great for many people with diabetes if there is a practitioner whom they can consult immediately over the phone or by email when they have a problem that they cannot solve themselves. It is helpful to have access to a psychologist with whom one may discuss the emotional aspects of living with this disease. But such small wonders do not show up in population statistics.

In short, the health of a population and that of the individuals who form a part of it do not improve in parallel. This leads to the so-called prevention paradox. If one wants to improve 'public health', more often than not caring for the individuals who need it turns out to be a bad investment. Take type 2 diabetes again. There is a range of care practices for people who have this disease. There are diets and drugs and patient groups and courses about how best to cope. Such care may improve people's individual situation in various ways, but it is mostly their so-called 'quality of life' that improves. However, even within populations of 'patients with type 2 diabetes', parameters such as mortality do not change all that much from such care.

Effects on the health of 'the population as a whole' are even harder to detect. Public health statistics are hardly affected by care for people with this disease, but a lot more by preventive measures. Diabetes statistics improve if people who are too heavy lose weight. The results are even better if something is done to prevent people of 'normal weight' putting on more weight. Public health does not improve as a result of caring for people who happen to have a disease. It improves from interventions that keep the healthy healthy. Individuals and populations need completely different types of care.

The hidden brave

In the logic of choice it is a tension. As long as individual health is at stake, the logic of choice wants individuals to make their own choices. How collective health is influenced by the choices people individually make is not taken into consideration. Maybe, as with a liberal economy, the hope is that it can be left to the workings of an invisible hand. However, when public health is at stake, another version of 'choice' is mobilised. For the invisible hand does not work all that well, and individuals who make their own choices do not automatically form healthy collectives. What is going on, do people lack 'information' or do they need to be told what is good for them? In one way or another, in the context of public health, 'choice' tends to no longer be appreciated as an ideal but accepted as a fact of life. Choosing is what people do. But they don't do it well enough, they should learn to make better choices. In order to improve public health, individuals are thus encouraged to 'choose to comply' with the rules set out by epidemiology.

In the logic of care, by contrast, there is a dilemma. What should we do: should care be given to individuals in need of care, or should we care for the health of the collective? In the first case, people with a disease get the care that fits their specific situation. In the second, it is more effective to influence the collective conditions under which we live in such a way that healthy people remain healthy. But while this dilemma presents itself in policy contexts, where decisions about collective action are made, it is not necessarily all that pressing in the consulting room, where individuals in need of care present themselves. If people come and complain, they get care. *If* they come and complain. Do all individuals in need of care indeed seek help? As things stand, the organisation of health care with its professionals who 'wait' for patients to appear in the consulting room, starts out from the assumption that people with a disease will seek help. And indeed, some do. But not everyone does. The crucial explanatory factor is not necessarily financial.

Interviewer: 'Are you the only person in your family with diabetes?' Lies Henstra: 'I guess so, but then again, the others never had themselves checked, but they may well have it too. My sister says: maybe I have it. She drinks and drinks. Not all that much, you know, but still. She could have diabetes. You can never tell.' In the Netherlands access to health care is easy. While insurance costs a lot of money, it tends to get paid. But even in this context, or so various surveys suggest, just about half of the patients with type 2 diabetes have been diagnosed. The other half remain hidden to care professionals until they have so many complications that they start to suffer badly. If they were to appear in the consulting room, they would be deemed to be 'in need of care'. But they don't go. Lies Henstra: 'I was sent to the eye specialist, because I have diabetes, and then they check your eyes. And they discovered that my eye pressure is too high. It was totally by chance that they discovered this. So I said: my husband may have high eye pressure too, but he never goes to see a doctor. Or my sister. We are all brave.'

What should we do about 'brave people'? As it is, they do not ask for care and therefore they do not receive care.[11] So long as you do not cause any trouble, nobody forces you to go to a consulting room. In the logic of care the dilemma is: should the health of the collective be given more attention, or is it better to concentrate on individual people in need of care? However, in between those two possibilities there is a gap. Who falls through? Professionals in a consulting room can do no more than attend to people who define themselves as being in need of care. People, that is, who take care of themselves. Health-care practices depend on active patients.

6 The good in practice

In this final chapter I weave together the arguments about the logic of choice and the logic of care that I have explored in previous chapters. In doing so, I begin by considering the topic of moral activity. Then I inquire into actorship. The articulation of what is implied in being an 'active patient' completes the argument of this book. Using as my case the treatment of, and life with, diabetes, I will have articulated a singular, specific, detailed version of the logic of care. I hope to have shown that care practices deserve to be appreciated and improved on their own terms. But how? What might a movement of active patients strive for? What might shared doctoring entail? Without going into details, I will offer some suggestions. And finally I will add some thoughts about further perspectives opened up by this analysis.

The logic of care articulated here originates from a highly specific site and situation. Even so, its implications may be wider. For instance, what follows if 'we' (whatever the term is made to mean: Westerners, modernists, humans) no longer take 'choice' to be crucial to who 'we' are, but downgrade it, and come to appreciate it as just one of our many activities? What follows if we no longer see 'making a choice' as a prerogative of specific people, but start to understand it as a characteristic of specific situations? Much would change as a consequence. Choice would no longer either be a defining fact of human life, or an achievement of Enlightenment. Instead, it would appear as an activity that may or may not be good to engage in in specific locations. Various questions follow, like where and when to organise situations of choice, and where and when other configurations might be more appropriate. For instance: configurations that resemble the treatment of and life with diabetes in and around hospital Z. Maybe, or so I would like to suggest, the logic of care deserves to be translated to a variety of other contexts.

Morality in action

By no means do I claim to stand on neutral ground, a place from where it is possible to judge which is better overall, the logic of choice or the logic of care. Instead, the analyses I have presented in this book so far, by contrasting the two logics, make it possible to compare the normativities they incorporate, their different grounds for evaluation. The 'good' relevant to each of them is different in kind – and so too is the 'bad'. While in the logic of choice autonomy and equality are good and oppression is bad, in the logic of care attentiveness and specificity are good and neglect is bad. Or the difference is more complex still. For not only does each logic define its own version of the good, each also has its own take on how to 'do' it. This is the topic that I would now like to address. How to serve the good actively, in practice? What are the crucial moral activities in the worlds that the two logics presuppose and help to create?

Let us begin again with the logic of choice. Its normativity is layered. There is a first explicitly normative layer: choice is a good, because it offers individuals autonomy; and equality is a good in that all individuals should have equal opportunities for making their own choices. There is a second layer, however, in which the logic of choice seeks to avoid making normative judgements. When it comes to the question as to which treatment, product, goal or life is best, the logic of choice provides no answer. Individuals are free to answer such questions for themselves. People may (or, in some versions of this logic, are required to) exercise their own judgement. The autonomy that (competent) individuals are entitled to within the logic of choice is precisely the autonomy of attaching their own value to just about everything (except autonomy). In the logic of choice making normative judgements is the moral activity *par excellence*, and it is this activity that this logic endorses.[1]

In this book I have examined customers as well as citizens. (The figure addressed by public health campaigns is a particular mixture of the two. I will talk about each figure separately and will leave out the added complexities that come with mixing them.) Customers and citizens have different styles of judging. In the (neo-classically shaped) market, individuals evaluate their options individually. Someone else may give them advice or try to seduce them with tempting advertisements, but in the end customers choose alone. Thus, the judgement entailed in that choice is not just individual but also private. In the market you do not need to justify your choices in public, it is enough to say 'I want this' – or to say nothing at all. Deciding what might be the best treatment, product, goal or way of life is a private matter. It is what everyone, or so the market logic has it, should do for themselves. In this respect citizens are different: they rule together. They coordinate their personal judgements in public, and to do so they engage in conversations about what it might be good to do. They do not hold on to private moralities, but seek to discuss ethics publicly. The privileged format for the continuing conversation between citizens is the public debate. In an ideal public debate participants clearly present the arguments that speak in favour of, and those that go against, particular options. The privileged method for the ethical discussion among citizens is to then balance the arguments, in the hope of reaching a collective verdict that, by taking all the relevant values into account, arrives at the best option. The ability of citizens to make their value judgements verbally explicit is a precondition for balancing values collectively in a discussion. Thus, while customers choose in silence and leave coordination to the market, citizens coordinate their choices with words.

In the logic of care a discussion where values are balanced so as to make ethically valid choices is not separated from other practices. This is not because value judgements are made in private. Something else is going on. In the logic of care, the crucial moral act is not making value judgements, but engaging in practical activities. There is only a single layer. It is important to do good, to make life better than it would otherwise have been. But what it is to do good, what leads to a better life, is not given before the act. It has to be established along the way. It may differ between lives, or between moments in a life. But, while it is impossible to ascertain in general what it is good to do, this does not mean that everyone has to figure it out for herself. The task of establishing what 'better' might be involves collectives. For instance, clinical epidemiological trials (which require the work of many researchers and even more patients) help to establish whether, say, a tight regulation of blood sugar levels now will or will not lead to fewer complications in due course. This is not to say that clinical trials define good care all by themselves. One may keep one's blood sugar levels stable by sticking to routines, or by persistently adjusting one's treatment to one's circumstances. Clinical trials cannot decide which of these brings along a better life. And, even if they can tell that your chances of complications diminish if you keep your blood sugar levels low, they cannot tell whether doing so is worth the trouble. Such matters can only be established by local doctoring. This still does not turn them into matters of choice. What you want is obviously relevant, but it is not decisive. For what you want most of all is not to have diabetes. But you do. Wishing your diabetes away does not help you to live with it. All kinds of other social and material practices that you are involved in rarely fit your wishes either. To some extent they may be changed, but where, and how? To find this out is a practical task, one that is experimental. So in the logic of care, defining 'good', 'worse' and 'better' does not precede practice, but forms part of it. A difficult part too. One that gives ample occasion for ambivalences, disagreements, insecurities, misunderstandings and conflicts. Nobody ever said that care would be easy.[2]

Establishing what 'better' might be is a difficult task and, once it seems to be clear, something is likely to change. Try again. On and on it goes. 'Good and bad' are never settled in the logic of care. A care team has to attend persistently to new twists, turns, problems, frictions and complications. This is demanding for professionals as well as for patients and requires that the consulting room is indeed used for consultation. Consultation is not debate. Good conversations in a consulting room do not take the shape of a confrontation between arguments, but are marked by an exchange of experiences, knowledge, suggestions, words of comfort. How have things been lately? What might be done differently and how might it be done? How do were adjust all the relevant elements in a patient's daily life to each other in the best possible way? Given the scope of the task, it is no wonder that in real existing care practices, care teams are rarely as free of friction as the logic of care would want them to be. As there is so much one has to do well, much may also go wrong. Just take the communication skills on which consultations depend: they are extensive. Pick the right words. Accept silences. Look at each other. Patients sit up straight or hunch their shoulders, a frightened or relieved look on their faces. Professionals smile, frown or search for something on their computer. Doctor and patient may lean together over the notebook with the results of blood sugar measurements. A nurse puts her hand on a patient's shoulder before she injects insulin. And then there are ever so many handshakes: consultations begin and end with one body touching another. Good communication is a crucial precondition for good care. It also is care in and of itself. It improves people's daily lives.

The conversation that helps to establish what might be good care, and what not, continues outside the consulting room. People with diabetes talk about their lives (disease included) with their relevant others, their relatives, their friends. Journalists conduct interviews and make documentaries so that care stories end up in newspapers, magazines and on television. Professionals publish striking experiences in professional journals. Social scientists assemble 'material' in slightly different ways in order to tell stories that shed new light on what goes on in the lives of people with a disease. All of this contributes to a public exchange that has a narrative rather than an argumentative style. The two styles are very different. While good arguments are unambiguous, good stories leave room for a variety of interpretations. While sound arguments should be clear and transparent, powerful stories work by evoking people's imagination, empathy and irritation. While conflicting arguments work against each other, conflicting stories tend to enrich each other. And while adding up arguments leads to a conclusion, adding on stories is more likely to be a way of raising ever more questions. How might what went wrong here be prevented elsewhere? How could we transport what was successful here to other sites and situations? And if there is nothing to be done, if nothing is likely to lead to any improvement, then stories may be a source of consolation.[3]

In the logic of care exchanging stories is a moral activity in and of itself. But moral activities do not restrict themselves to talk, to verbal exchanges. They also come in physical forms. As a part of their self-care, patients measure their blood sugar levels, eat wisely, exercise and inject their insulin. The other members of the care team also put in physical effort. Doctors pump up a cuff to measure blood pressure. They touch you to find out if your skin is hardening where you inject your insulin. Nurses gently make a fold in your skin as they administer injections. And collective, public investment in care is physical as well. At some point someone cut open dogs and removed their pancreases in order to learn more about diabetes. In doing so, he not only put his job at stake but also sacrificed the lives of the dogs. Someone else volunteered to be the first person to be injected with insulin. This person obviously hoped to live longer, but at the same time put herself at risk. Dogs without pancreases thrived on such injections, but nobody knew for certain if a human patient would do so too, or if she would die on the spot.[4] It has happened time and time again in the history of diabetes care: innovators put mental, emotional and physical effort into developing new drugs, technologies and techniques. A few patients dared to try these experimental treatments. By taking the risks involved on their shoulders, they related to future patients, giving them an invaluable gift. Relating to others physically is an inextricable part of collectively investing in care.[5]

Innovation is important to the logic of choice as well. Here, however, it is not a moral activity. Instead, researchers are supposed to be impartial. They develop modest means that serve ends that have been established elsewhere. Good means are not morally good, instead they are effective. Technologies are meant to create opportunities, not obligations. If they happen to agree with the ends, potential users may choose to use them, but they do not need to. There is no obligation, or so the logic of choice has it. But is this true? Once you step into the logic of care all this seems to be a striking simplification. Innovations that care are never neutral: they cannot be. Since they are made to contribute to improving lives, they incorporate some notion of what counts as an 'improvement'. What is more: innovations tend to be morally complex. Take injectable insulin. History books say that the inventor of this novelty was after personal gain (a better job, money, fame), but this selfish investment does not devalue his invention. Indeed, it is precisely because injectable insulin improved the lives of so many people, that its inventor was also able to gain from it personally. Then there is the innovation itself. Is injectable insulin merely a modest means? Does it simply present people with an opportunity, take it or leave it? Obviously, people with diabetes can decide against injecting insulin. If they are not under age, demented, or declared to be of unsound mind, nobody can force treatment upon them. But this does not mean that insulin is modest and subjects itself to our ends. Instead it has changed the moral landscape. Prior to the existence of manufactured insulin, dying from diabetes at a young age was a tragic fate. Nowadays, if you happen to have diabetes and refuse to inject insulin, this amounts to committing suicide. As a result of manufacturing insulin, 'not injecting' has become a lethal act, and hence a moral activity. This is what technologies do. They shift both the practical and the moral frameworks of our existence.

Do they do so in a good way? This remains to be seen – but how? In the logic of choice establishing what is good is a matter of weighing and balancing. In order to make a judgement about what to do, you gather as many arguments for and against this or that course of action as you can, and weigh them up. Sometimes a new argument pops up later and makes you change your mind. But inevitably a more or less balanced judgement, the best judgement you can make then and there, precedes action. This is different in the logic of care. Here, action does not come after moral closure has been achieved: action itself is moral. But it is never comfortable. You do your best, but it is impossible to predict how an attempt to do good will work out in practice. Take insulin again. If it had been impossible to manufacture insulin on an industrial scale, it is quite likely that over the course of time more effort would have been spent on the development of technologies to protect or repair the pancreas. Along the way a lot of people would have died at an early age, but, who knows, the resulting treatment might have been better. As it is, most people with diabetes who have access to insulin are grateful. This drug keeps them alive, while without it they would die. Worldwide, many people die of diabetes. Manufactured insulin is expensive, and depends on an extensive infrastructure. And while insulin is life-saving, it is not a cure. Regulating an internal feedback system from the outside is never entirely successful. What should we do if problems emerge? More injections; more exercise; a different diet; another doctor; fewer injections; less exercise; therapy to deal with fear of injections; or no longer trying so terribly hard. In the logic of care uncertainty is chronic, and additional arguments cannot hope to alter this. You do what you can, you try and try again. You doctor, but you have no control. And ultimately the result is not glorious: stories about life with a disease do not end with everybody 'living happily ever after'. They end with death. Just like the stories about other lives.

The logic of care has no separate moral sphere. Because 'values' intertwine with 'facts', and caring itself is a moral activity, there is

drawn into health care, it does not finally make space for a 'self' that was already there. Instead, something is being asked from us. Situations are being reshaped in such a way that choices are called for and we are called upon to make those choices. The promise is that this will finally free us, patients, from the passivity in which professionals have kept us trapped. By making choices, or so the logic of choice claims, we become the masters of our own lives. This promise of mastery, however, hides what it costs to reshape the world in such a way that 'situations of choice' are created. The logic of care has different strengths and different limits. My point is not that it is always intrinsically better. It is rather that it deserves to be better attended to. Not because, in its turn, it serves our true selves. The logic of care is again demanding, but what it asks from us is different. No, it does not ask patients to meekly agree with the prescriptions of professionals. It wants us to be active. What, then, is an active patient?

In the logic of choice an actor is someone who makes decisions. In order to make decisions actors have to consider the relevant arguments and weigh up the advantages and disadvantages of the options available. This is not easy and all but impossible if you have a fever, are in coma, or if you are shaking with fear. But if you have a chronic disease, you may well be able to mobilise your healthy part to make your choices. So you choose. What follows from your choice, for better or worse, is your responsibility. You have to carry it on your shoulders. Given that making choices is difficult, it is no surprise that the question who has and who lacks the ability to choose receives so much attention. In the logic of care ability is more fluid in kind. This is not to say that the logic of care makes life easy for us. It again asks us to take a lot upon ourselves. Not guilt this time, but a wide range of activities. In the logic of care actors do things: they inject insulin, avoid a hypo by feeling or measuring and counteracting it, and they calculate what they eat. But no actor needs to act alone: in the logic of care the action moves around. One moment you care and the next you are taken care of. Care tasks are shared in varying ways. They also change. Something is done – and when it doesn't work the crucial question is not whose fault it was, but what to try next. In the logic of care the fact that the patient has a disease affects what needs to be done, but it does not absolve the patient from playing an active part in the doing. You do not have to do everything by yourself. You cannot: even doctors with diseases need professional care.[6] But you always do something. If you are unable to inject your own insulin, a nurse does it for you. However, instead of fighting when she approaches you with a needle, you allow her to inject you. You may be unable to calculate what you eat. Then you follow the instructions of the dietician, but you are still the one to chew, swallow and digest your food. If even that is too much for you and you are being fed artificially, you remain an actor. As long as you are alive your cells burn sugar.

In the logic of care being an actor is primarily a practical matter. This does not mean that nobody ever needs to make choices. Instead, in this logic 'making a choice' appears as yet another practical task. Take the choice 'shall I play sport seriously or not?' This depends on more than arguments. Being able to balance your values is not enough, you also have to be able to balance your energy. Thus, as a part of making this choice, you have to figure out if you can get yourself to eat on time, measure, adapt your insulin dose. Hours after your football match or your jogging hour, your blood sugar level may still drop: can you watch out for that? Freedom is hard work. If you want to walk in the mountains, that is fine, but just wanting it is not enough. You have also to engage in the practical work that such walking depends on. And this includes making many small, practical choices. If you sit down to measure and your blood sugar level appears to be 3 mmol/l, you simply need to eat. But what if it is 5, 6 or 7 but you still have an hour of climbing ahead? On and on it goes. These days people with diabetes are no longer obliged to stick to routines, but can choose to have one, two or three sandwiches for lunch. But many people (and not just people with diabetes) tend to avoid choices like these. For figuring out what to do next, day by day, minute by minute, is draining. So instead, most of us experiment with daily life until we have established acceptable routines. An evening meal by six-thirty every day. Or two sandwiches for lunch on weekdays and three on a Saturday (before playing football or going to jog). In practice, routines consume a lot less energy than making fresh choices over and over again.[7]

In the logic of choice actors make judgements in order to choose. Thus they take a distance. It is, after all, easiest to judge something outside yourself: a blood sugar monitor, syringes or an insulin pen. You may label these as accurate or inaccurate, user-friendly or cumbersome. At least you may do so when these objects are foreign to you. It gets more difficult if you have been using a device for some time, for then it has become 'a part of you'. It is hard to judge something that is a part of yourself as if from a distance. It is even harder to make judgements about your own life. Health-care researchers ask us to do this. We are supposed to tick boxes on questionnaires on a scale of 1 to 5. How much does your diabetes bother you, 0 (not at all), 3 (a little) or 5 (a lot)? The numbers are added up, and the total is meant to represent our 'quality of life'. In the logic of care judging one's life does not make sense. You are inside your life, you live it. You cannot disentangle yourself from it and establish its quality from a distance. If ever a patient were to say in the consulting room 'Doctor, my quality of life is low', the reaction of the doctor would not be to note this in the patient's file as a fact. Instead, the doctor would wonder what might be done about it. She would ask: 'Tell me, what exactly is going wrong?' Or: 'How can I help you?' In the logic of care life is not to be taken for a fact, but as a task. What would your friends say if you told them that your 'quality of life' is poor? They might sympathise, but wouldn't they then ask: 'Well, what are you going to do about it?' Rather than taking you for a spectator of your life, they expect you to play the leading part in it. Thus, in the logic of care it is not the noun that is crucial, *life* (an object that may be judged), but rather the verb, *to live* (an activity of which we are the subjects).

In the logic of choice actors are emancipated. They have liberated themselves from patriarchal rulers. The glorification of freedom that comes with this makes it difficult to recognise the activities of active patients. For the patients addressed by the logic of care are not free. However, neither do they depend primarily on their doctors and nurses (patriarchal or otherwise). People with diabetes depend first and foremost on their insulin. That is their lifeline. As is the food they eat; and the glucagon others inject for them if a deep hypo has set in. Independence is nice, but not to the extent that it is killing. At the same time others depend on the ever so dependent patients: their colleagues, partners, elderly parents and young children. And so, too, do the professionals in their care team. If patients turn passive, professionals cannot do anything either. It may be possible to rule others or make their choices for them, but it is impossible to take care of people who do not take care of themselves. It cannot be done. If people are brave and do not seek help, nobody can give it to them. If a patient at home stops injecting her insulin, the doctor and the nurse won't even know. Thus, however dependent patients may be, their care depends in the first place on their own activities. Patients with diabetes even do a lot that was formerly done by professionals. In other parts of health care it is nurses who give intramuscular injections. People with diabetes do this themselves. In other contexts it is laboratory technicians who measure relevant blood levels. People with diabetes do this themselves. Adjusting the dose of drugs is traditionally a doctor's task. Quite a few active patients with diabetes do this themselves as well. When they break with their routines, they inject a few units more or less, as need be.

Despite all this activity, as a patient you do not control the world. The world is not obedient. Blood sugar levels, eyes, other people, food, machines, what have you: everything behaves unpredictably. No matter how hard you try to tame the various aspects of your life, in the end they are irreducibly wild. You may succeed or you may fail: either way you have to live with it. Thus active patients need to be both active and able to let go. They need to actively take their care into their own hands and yet to let go of whatever it is they cannot tame. So there it is again, the most difficult thing that the logic of care demands of us: being tenacious as well as adaptable. Professionals take years to develop a clinical attitude: they are trained to respond actively to their patients' suffering, while at the same time accepting quietly that their efforts may fail. Active patients have a far more difficult task: they have to be energetic as well as resigned about their own suffering.[8] It is not to be underestimated, this huge emotional and practical effort. And yet it is likely to be better than the illusion that you may yet control the world. For dreams of control do not make you happy, they make you neurotic. And one way or the other they end in disappointment.

The logic of care is not better or worse than the logic of choice always and everywhere. I do not want to make general claims. But this much I assert: the logic of care is definitely better geared to living with a diseased and unpredictable body. Therefore the patient movement would be wise not to dismiss this logic too lightly. It should instead examine it, adapt it, fiddle with it, push and pull it, alter it, as and where this seems right. The logic of care as I articulate it here is not something to solidify or cast in stone. Not at all! It is fluid and adaptable. But it is a good place to start from since, instead of addressing only the part of us that is healthy, it takes us seriously as we are, diseases and all. It seeks to nourish our bodies; respects the collectivities to which we belong; reacts forgivingly to our failures; and stubbornly strives for improvement, even if things keep on going wrong; though not beyond an (un-)certain limit, for in the end it will let go. Although it is difficult to relate to one's own suffering in a clinical way, learning to combine being active with being receptive does more than strengthening our capacity to care. For the ability to let go actively not only makes suffering easier to bear. It is also a pre-condition for experiencing pleasure.[9]

Improving health care

That the logic of choice and the logic of care are so profoundly different begs the question as to what happens when these two modes of thinking and acting get mixed together – as they do in real life. The possible interferences are many. Indeed, what has happened in those places where patient choice has been introduced into health care is highly variable. Only detailed empirical studies of different sites and situations are likely to give insight into the various kinds of interferences. I do not doubt that some of these will prove to be surprisingly creative, and better for living than the 'pure' forms I have distilled from the messiness of hospital practice. And yet I have tried to articulate the logic of care here in an undiluted form in the hope of strengthening it. For no matter how loudly the wonders of patient choice are celebrated, I am not so optimistic. My worry is that, with the introduction of patient choice, many other things get fixed as well: the circumstances in which we make our choices; the alternatives between which we may choose; the boundaries around the 'care products' we may or may not opt for; and so on. Fixing all of these things would frustrate doctoring, as it would make it even more difficult to attune the various viscous variables relevant in care to each other. What is more, 'choice' comes with many hierarchical dichotomies that are foreign to 'care': active versus passive; health versus disease; thinking versus action; will versus fate; mind versus body. Bringing these dichotomies into play is not going to improve the lives of people with a disease, if only because they end up time and again on the wrong side of the divide.

However, that it is possible to articulate a logic of care that gives words to what 'good care' is about does not imply that as things stand most health-care practices are good. A lot of them are not – not good enough. Actually, the requirements for good care are exceedingly difficult to meet. And there is much (scientific fashion; managerial ambition; economic pulls and pushes; and yes, careless professionals, too) that works against the realisation of good care in practice. Thus articulating 'good care' is not a way of describing the facts, of telling about the world as it is. Nor is it an evaluation, a (positive) judgement of care practices. Instead, it is an intervention. Articulating the logic of care is an attempt to contribute to improving health care on its own terms, in its own language. A language in which the main emphasis is not on autonomy and the right to decide for oneself, but on daily life practices and attempts to make these more liveable through inventive doctoring. In care-specific terms, care is bad when people are being neglected. When there is not enough time to listen. When physical parameters are isolated from their context; when patients' daily lives are not taken into consideration. When patients are left to their own devices and have to face the complex (and sometimes impossible) task of combining the divergent instructions given to them by different specialists. When professionals fail to carry out careful experiments, but hastily follow protocols instead, or – even worse – lazily fall back on old habits. In care-specific terms, care is bad when the measurement of a few discrete parameters displaces attention from the sometimes painful and always complicated intricacies of day-to-day life with a disease.

When in interviews – or elsewhere – patients complain about bad health care, they may mention that they were not given a choice, but more often they talk about neglect. They describe how their particular stories or personal experiences were not attended to. They would have appreciated more interaction and more support. Or they say that there was nothing they could do and not enough was done for them. This feeling of being deserted becomes tangible in Mr Gradus's story about the time his insulin pump stopped working. He had recently moved house and his new doctor was not familiar with his particular pump, so Mr Gradus phoned his old hospital. He was put through to one person after another. Nobody was able to give him advice. Finally, he got hold of someone who suggested he contact the manufacturer. Meanwhile he had become worried about his blood sugar levels. What should he do: eat something now, since it was getting quite late? He did not want a hypo. But what if his blood sugar levels were to soar when he ate? He did not know what to do. He no longer had a syringe and the insulin to go with it. He did not have a pen. When he finally managed to get hold of the manufacturer, he was told that his pump was out of date. Spare parts or replacement pumps were no longer available. What should he do? Whom should he turn to now? That desolate feeling of being abandoned has stayed with him, and he still speaks about it years later. The point is not that others boss you about, but that nobody cares. A hole opens up and you fear that you will fall right through it.

Overall there are too many holes. Even people with a place to go to may find that there is nobody there who listens to them properly and takes what they have to say into account. Nobody who is interested in their experiences with uncertainty, fear, shame, loneliness and the never-ending pressure of having to take care of themselves. Even their experiences with physical issues like unstable blood sugar levels are not really attended to. In the hospital where I did my field work, one of the physicians at some point asked all the patients of the diabetes outpatient clinic to complete a short questionnaire about any 'hypoglycaemic incidents' they had encountered during the last few weeks. The laboratory cannot measure hypos retrospectively: they leave no detectable trace in your blood. But patients remember most hypos vividly: these are nasty experiences. Answering the questionnaires, the patients reported many more 'incidents' than the doctors had expected. Apparently these doctors did not ask their patients about their hypos as a matter of routine in the consulting room. They had read the clinical trials that say that tight regulation helps to prevent long-term complications. But they had failed to observe that in the daily life of their own patients tight regulation leads to lots of hypos. An inquisitive researcher, a questionnaire and a number of patients willing to fill it out were needed to make this visible. The researcher's conclusion was that more fine-tuning and increased attentiveness to the specificities of every single patient were urgently required. This would be better for people's daily lives (which are disrupted by hypos) and their bodies were likely to benefit as well (hypos cause brain damage). The researcher in question published her findings, but where were they heard? And what other daily experiences with diseases and their treatments are left unexamined?

The logic of care wants professionals not to blindly apply the

results of clinical trials, but to translate them carefully. That is doctoring. Potentially helpful technologies should be locally fine-tuned.
This requires that the doctoring be shared. For treatments can only
be adjusted properly if the experiences of patients are carefully
attended to. The terms I just used are all normative. The logic of care
wants these things to happen; says that they should be done; or
requires them. In practice, however, it doesn't always work this
way. Care doesn't always meet the standards of good care implied in
the logic of care. To try to make it do so would be to improve care
on its own terms. This is first and foremost a task for professional
practice; it has to do with what is done in the consulting room. Along
with this, it has to do with the organisational conditions that allow
consulting rooms to be configured in one way rather than another.
Here, I will not attend to those organisational contexts, but move on
to another precondition for work in the consulting room. Lived
reality also needs to be better incorporated into scientific research. It
is here, after all, that new interventions are developed and assessed.[10]
What is done with and to diseases in scientific research – and to our
lives with them? It is quite remarkable that so much public attention
is given to the (political) representation of the patient's will, and so
little to the (scientific) representation of patient bodies and patient
lives. As if what we might want does not depend to a large extent on
the matters of fact gathered about us. As it is, such facts all too often
take the form of correlations between parameters, measured in large
numbers. Ideally, research projects measure the parameters that are
most relevant for patients' daily lives. But this ideal is rarely met.
Often, parameters are measured because they are easy to measure, or
because they happen to be the parameters most frequently mentioned
in the literature. Even well-selected parameters are necessarily
selected early in the research process. Researchers who want to find
out whether or not an intervention works have to begin by defining
their criteria for 'working'. However, the unexpected effects of
interventions only begin to surface later on. They will only be
noticed if someone is on the lookout for them.

The scientific tradition that is currently most prominent in health
care – that of clinical epidemiology – has not been designed to deal
with the unexpected effects of interventions. Tracing these requires
that one be open to surprises. Since unforeseen events cannot be
foreseen and unidentified variables cannot be counted, other research

methods are needed to learn more about them. Promising among these are the clinical interview and the case report. In good clinical interviews patients are granted time and space to talk about what they find striking, difficult or important. Their diverse and surprising experiences are carefully attended to. Case reports, in their turn, are stories about remarkable events. They make these events transportable, so that others may learn from them. Since case reports did not fit with rationalist fashions, their format has hardly changed over the past few decades: it begs to be improved. By tradition, case histories were written by doctors, about events that happened to individual patients, for an audience of medical colleagues. As we move towards 'shared doctoring', each of these elements can be adapted. Next to doctors, others might also author case histories: other (health-care) professionals, patients, onlookers. Anthropologists and journalists (in their own different ways) may experiment with stories told in multiple voices, gathering the experiences of a wide range of people. Instead of only the individual with a disease, larger collectives may also be topicalised in case histories. The intended audience may be broadened as well, from medical colleagues to all the rest of us. Moreover, where case histories traditionally moved freely between blood values and fears, pain receptors and workloads, they can be made to incorporate yet more (f)actors: insurance arrangements, the food industry, the accessibility of local swimming pools, and so on. The difficult but much loved demented partner. Good walking shoes and socks. The art is to track down and attune to the specificities that are relevant.

However, when it comes to improving care practices, publicly telling rich stories is not enough. We also need spaces where it is possible to act in new ways, experimental spaces. Clinical trials were developed in response to innovative research by the pharmaceutical industry. They were designed to monitor the drugs the industry developed. Was it safe to allow these drugs onto the market? Was it worthwhile spending collective insurance money on them?[11] But in other contexts, where it is not so obvious what to separate out from the care process as something to be sold, it is not obvious what exactly to measure. What is more: who should take on the role of innovator? Industry may develop drugs and apparatus that might change hands. But who is likely to develop caring interventions that do not have a marketable product at their centre? Here, there is room for improvement: creative practitioners (physicians, nurses, dieticians, physiotherapists, patients and patient groups) need time, money and space to experiment with innovations for daily care practices. Good local findings then need to be spread to other places. As it is, local inventions about the shaping of daily life with diabetes are being made even if there is little infrastructure for this. They deserve to be allowed to travel, but how? How do we best shift arrangements that help people to live well with their disease to other patients in other, different sites and situations?

But not only is there a lot to learn from practices that work well. Failures, too, are instructive. The traditional case history often dealt with failures, because these surprised the doctor who reported on them almost as much as miraculous recoveries. What is more: if others were told about them, they might avoid making the same mistakes. In this light, it is remarkable that current accountability practices require professionals to prove that they do well. Professionals are constantly required to praise themselves. Here are the evaluation forms, account for what you have been doing! There is no room for doubt, self-criticism, or difficult questions. However, improvement begins with the recognition that something needs to be improved. That not everything is as it should be. It fits with the logic of care to attend to frictions and problems. To acknowledge that some things do not work well, no matter how well intended they may be. This suggests an entirely different accountability practice. Not one in which everyone has to say how wonderful they are, but one in which people feel safe enough to examine what in their practices tends to go wrong and why. This can be done in various collectives: with people who share the same expertise; or with people involved with the same ward, from professors to cleaners; on the level of a hospital, a neighbourhood, or a nation; among professionals; among patients; among all the people caring (whether as professional or as patient) for the same disease; and so on. So long as nobody is pushed onto the defensive, it is also possible to allow critical outsiders with a fresh, keen eye into care institutions. They might look for frictions and problems, not in order to detect and punish the guilty, but in order to learn. In the consulting room (or so the idealised logic of care that I have presented here implies), professionals and patients engage in the shared doctoring that is necessary to improve what does not work well in a patient's daily life. Something similar could be done in other sites and situations, in a variety of ever-changing collectives. Thus we could share the improvement of health-care practices too.

In all this, the criteria that differentiate between good and bad care are not given in advance. Defining improvement is an integral part of the activity of improving. The reflection required cannot be separated out from trying to establish in practice what can be done. There are obviously limits to the fluidity of these criteria-in-the-making. Most of the time death is a presence felt in the background of diabetes care and most of the time it is a 'bad'. It is to be avoided. This sets limits to the experiments one might want to engage in. Health, the other limit, is not on offer: diabetes cannot be cured. In between these two alternatives, the question of how to improve daily life, or how best to live it, is multifaceted and complicated enough to make it worthwhile to keep on tinkering. What is good: a longer life, or one lived more intensely? Is it possible to keep on driving, or better to leave your job? Do you stick to your identity as a food lover, or try to learn to postpone gratification? Nothing will ever be perfect. But you keep on trying. And while you do so, even death does not always remain something bad to avoid. At some point, it may come as a relief. Sooner or later, it is inevitable, death. So what do we die from?

Instead of wrestling with all these questions individually, at isolated moments when we cannot avoid difficult choices, it might be better to address them collectively. Out loud. Not only inside, but also outside the consulting room. Let us doctor, and thus, in careful ways, experiment with our own lives. And let us tell each other stories. Case histories. Public life deserves to be infused with rich stories about personal events. Private events should not be hidden behind the desire to be free. In fact, the story-telling I advocate is already happening. Journalists, patient activists, social scientists and others too, present us with an avalanche of stories about living with disease. I do not claim to be proposing something new here, but rather seek to raise the status of 'telling stories'. Rather than a matter of 'merely' sharing private experiences, telling stories is a form of public coordination. It is part of how we govern ourselves and each other. For only by persistently posing the questions of life and death out loud may we hope to incorporate the best answers into the technologies, the drugs, and the health-care organisations that, whether we want it or not, we inevitably share.[12]

Translations

The aim of this book is not to pass judgement. I do not seek to criticise health care in general and neither do I want to celebrate it. The
point is rather to contribute to its improvement. But how? I did not
develop the much desired blood sugar monitor that accurately measures sugar levels without obliging people to prick their fingers. I have
not helped to set up a new clinic. I did not invent new conversational
techniques. I have not assembled creative ideas about how best to live
with diabetes. And I am certainly not about to formulate ethical rules
about what others should and should not do with their technologies,
their skills or their lives. While the grant that allowed me to work on
this book was meant for research that would lead to policy recommendations that might be implemented tomorrow, I carefully abstain
from giving such recommendations. Even the stories I have told here
are too few and fragmented to contribute seriously to the vivid,
ongoing public conversation about life with diseases that I advocate.
Instead, my contribution has been of a different kind. In this book I
have articulated the (all too silent) logic that is incorporated in good
care. I have tried to put it into words so as to help in shifting it from
private consulting rooms to public discussions. I offer no solutions,
but language. The contribution this book tries to make is theoretical.

The logic of care itself is first and foremost practical. It is concerned with actively improving life. Until recently it did not have to
defend itself, or to be defended, in so many words. Not so long ago
health care and the logic it incorporated were beyond doubt, unques-
tionably good. This is why, back in the 1960s and 1970s, social scientists and philosophers started to raise questions about health care.
They critically explored the bad effects of good intentions. They
questioned medical power and unmasked 'health' as a problematic
ideal. I do not deny the value of that endeavour. It shook things up. It
interfered with the arrogance of far too many medical professionals.
However, if criticism goes on and on it becomes mechanical.
Whether it is true or not, it is no longer engaging. It tells us nothing
new. To shake things up again and in new ways we now need other
strategies. But what strategies, and where do we find them? Our
theoretical frameworks seem to be too exclusively adapted to the
task of 'criticism'. They unmask. They tend not to explore or build
ideals but to undermine them. Thus, the question as to what 'good

care' might be was left to rationalists seeking to serve goods such as 'efficacy' and 'efficiency'. But what might be good for patients, which ways of living with a disease might be better than their alternatives? Without a language to address these questions collectively, answering them was left to everyone individually. Let people choose for themselves. That the social sciences and philosophy did not seek to praise some version of 'good care' created a vacuum. It is partly due to this vacuum that 'autonomous choice', an ideal that originally took shape in quite different contexts, so rapidly conquered health care.

Recently, however, the tide seems to be turning. Choice is being subjected to doubt, while care has received positive attention.[13] This book is part of that turn and seeks to contribute to it. But how far does it reach, the logic of care presented here? Where it comes from is easy to point out. A lot of what I learned from earlier studies (my own and those of others that I read about) has seeped into this project. But, in order to be specific and precise, I have taken a single, particular case as my lead. The 'care' articulated here, is the care for, and by, people with diabetes in the Netherlands at the beginning of the twenty-first century. And even that is putting it too broadly: I have skipped over many variants. This study in no way resembles a survey or an overview. So, if you were to study a different case, the 'care' you might come to articulate would be different too. For example: people with diabetes engage in an impressive amount of self-care, but people with dementia do not. Indeed, it is central to their disease that they gradually lose the ability to look after themselves. Thus the demands on family, friends and professionals in the two cases of care are quite different, as are the experiences of patients. Or, another point of contrast, while living with diabetes requires endless doctoring, living with cancer generates more obvious and irreversible bifurcation points. Points at which one is made to consider whether it would be better to accept the unpleasant side-effects of treatment, or to let go and die instead. Framed in this way, these are inescapable choices, dilemmas that cannot be tinkered with. So the logic of care is not a single configuration. I have presented just one version of it here. If we shift diagnosis, specialisms, hospitals, financial systems, religions, rules and regulations, opportunities for employment, languages, social relations and so on (the possibilities are endless) then some aspects of this care version will remain relevant while others do not. A book like this is written in the hope that its readers will not absorb it passively, but use it actively. So there is work left to do for you, reader. Which elements of the logic of care articulated here fit with the contexts that you find yourself in, and which do not? What stays the same, what alters? What remains worthwhile and what does not? This book provides no answers to that; you will have to think about those questions yourself. I wish you good luck.

When transported to other sites and situations, the logic of care articulated here will have to be translated. Many translations are possible and it is impossible to anticipate them all. But I would like to make one final claim: the logic of care is not only relevant to health care. Its implications and its relevance are far wider. A first reason for that is that the very existence of a logic of care implies that 'the West' does not fit into the framework liberal social theories try to fit it in. Such theories oppose freedom with submission. They hold rationality to be a glorious human trait, or better still, an achievement of Enlightenment. They presume that societies in 'the West' consist of free individuals who make rational choices; privately at home and on the market, and publicly in the context of the state. Let us bracket for now the question as to whether or not this is true for customers and citizens: for patients it is certainly not. Not because patients are submitted to others who rule over them, but because they are taken care of and take care of themselves. Caring activities, shared in various ways, criss-cross the boundary between private and public. Doctoring eludes the rational fantasies of control as it involves fragile bodies and not quite predictable machines. These transgressive traits imply that care practices are heterotopias to Western philosophy. A heterotopia is a place that is *other*. It allows one to see old issues with new eyes; and to listen with strange ears to what seemed to speak for itself.[14] This specific heterotopia, however, that of care, is not elsewhere, but within. It offers contrasts that help us to understand more about 'choice', while they also reveal where 'choice' hits its limits.

Though it certainly infuses many practices, the logic of choice does not inform everything that happens in 'the West'. Life with diabetes escapes from it. But it is unlikely that it is only life with diabetes that does this. What else exceeds the logic of choice? Educating. Farming. Sailing. Making music. Fighting. Building.

Filming. Raising children. Making television programmes. Engaging in scientific research. Loving. Cooking. Cleaning. Writing. They all have their own style; or rather varied styles. Numerous logics wait to be explored.[15] So this is my claim. In this book the province that took itself for the world has (once more) been put back into a small corner. 'The West' holds no universal insights, valid everywhere, that it can ground in rationality. It does not bask in the triumphs of Enlightenment. If 'the West' is anything, then it is an amalgam of highly divergent ways of thinking and acting. A heterogeneous assemblage of logics; of co-existing languages irreducible to each other; interwoven with disparate practices.[16] A conglomerate of contradictions.

But, while the various logics that inform our practices clash with one another, they are also interdependent. Without farmers, customers have nothing to eat. Without care, citizens die when they get a nasty disease. Without homes, writers cannot sleep. And, while each logic originates in a specific site and situation, they all move about. They go from one place to another. The logic of choice has moved into health care, bringing along, or brought along by, informed consent forms, litigation, advertisements aimed at patients, and the slogan 'It's your own choice.' My point is not that it is impossible, or generally bad, for logics to move. Rather, I question whether, in this particular case, it is desirable. The logic of choice, or so I claim, does not accord very well with life with a disease. But logics need not necessarily stay where they come from, as if the place where they originated was the only one where they belong. Take the logic of care. With this book I want to help to strengthen and revitalise this logic. But, if I argue that health care deserves to be improved on its own terms, this does not mean that these terms only make sense inside health care. They might (be made to) move around.[17] But where? And what would happen if the logic of care were indeed transported to other sites and situations?

It is not obvious. In many circumstances it may well be difficult to be as rigorously specific as good care requires. And while general rules (for instance those favoured by the law) are never quite specific enough in particular situations, they have the advantage of being easy to use: they can be called upon by those who feel treated in an unfair way. That there are no fixed variables in the logic of care generates the possibility of fluid adaptation, but it also implies

that there is nothing fixed to hold on to. That the logic of care takes
failures to be an unavoidable part of life makes it difficult to establish when some limit has been reached, or, worse, transgressed, and
it is appropriate to be angry. Is there space left for 'criticism' within
the logic of care? And it is all well and good to ask people to keep
on going, tenaciously but not obsessively, energetically but not
excessively so. But where should these people find the courage and
the energy that this requires? Doctoring is highly demanding and
especially so when your own suffering is at stake. What is more: in
health care there is a tradition of paid professionals who specialise in
(their various variants of) doctoring. They collectively foster their
knowledge and their professional ethos. They may be called upon to
support lay people in their care work. In many other areas of social
life, such professionals are absent. More generally, one may wonder
what kinds of institutional conditions are needed for care to flourish.

These are serious limitations, or even objections, to moving the
logic of care about. But then again: the list of elements from the logic
of care that might be inspiring for practices elsewhere is at least as
striking. Take the raw honesty about failure and misery. Disease,
death, suffering, problems: care begins by facing these. They are not
kept out of the equation as mere noise, nor taken to be offensive
transgressions to be avoided at all costs. They are not marginalised.
Instead they are talked about and tinkered with, they are attended to
and subjected to doctoring. In that process pseudo-certainty is not
invoked: there is no need for it. In the logic of care doubt does not
preclude action. The attitude is experimental: you interact with the
world, while seeking what brings improvement and what does not.
This may well be helpful in many circumstances. Lack of water, lack
of food, lack of clean air, lack of space. Regardless of whether the
lives at stake are those of humans, animals, plants or ecosystems.[18]
Try and try again. There is no need for the excessive optimism that
will inevitably end in disappointment, but neither is there an excuse
for fatalism. Give up dreams of perfection or control, but keep on
trying. But who is addressed; who should keep on trying; who should
act? The answer is: everyone and everything. For in the logic of care
actors do not have fixed tasks. The 'we' who does the doing may
shift. There is no need to distinguish between scientific, commercial,
political and other (collective) actors in an attempt to establish who
may, or should, do this or that. In the logic of care the action is more

Acknowledgements

In the spring of 2005 I presented earlier versions of several of the chapters of this book to academic audiences in Seattle, Santa Cruz and Claremont, USA. A few weeks before I was due to visit, the local organiser in Santa Cruz emailed me to ask if I could send a written version of my presentation for the benefit of the person who was going to act as a commentator. Sure, I wrote back, I have a text and I can send it, so long as the commentator reads Dutch. At that time this book only existed in a rough Dutch version, and I like to tame my frustrations about the untransportability of my mother tongue by teasing native speakers of English with their inability to read it. Their shame about the asymmetry (I read and write their language!) is at least somewhat comforting. However, on this occasion I was beaten. The next day I opened my mail box and found a message from a then Santa Cruz PhD, David Machledt. In Dutch. A few errors maybe, but nothing I could not easily understand. Yes, he wrote, send it, I'll try. And so he did.

So for David Machledt I would not have needed to translate this text into English. He gave good comments on a draft of chapter 3 (thanks, Dave!) and he would have managed to read the rest in Dutch as well. However, the interest of the other people in those audiences encouraged me to try to reach them too. So I would like to thank Janelle Taylor, Nancy Chen and Marianne de Laet for invitations and mediations. And Lisa Diedrich, Rebecca Young and Rayna Rapp for giving me the occasion to get questions and comments from Stony Brook and New York audiences a year later. And let me thank Michi Knecht and Stefan Beck and their other guests for an inspiring international workshop in a small castle near Berlin.

I presented an overview of the argument laid out here at a

gathering at the Open University, in Milton Keynes, UK. Steve Hinchliffe and Nick Bingham, who organised it, and everyone else who was present gave truly helpful responses. For their criticism on an earlier English-language draft, and for their encouragements, I also thank Nicolas Dodier, Arthur Frank, David Healy, Tiago Moreira, Ingunn Moser, Vicky Singleton and Steve Woolgar. Simon Cohn kindly commented on the penultimate version. Crucial among the many questions that arose during the project of translating, was whether the Dutch expression 'logica van het zorgen' would best be translated into 'logic of caring' (to stress that we are dealing with a verb here, and a process) or into 'logic of care' (a nicer sounding phrase that makes for a better contrast with 'logic of choice'). I thank Nick Bingham for taking that decision for me – as well as for his careful attention to senses and sentences in the rest of this book.

A first translation of the entire text was made by Ron Peek of Peek Language Services. He did a great job in an incredibly short time for which I am most grateful. However, a text like this depends on meticulous details in its writing. It was interesting to see how often wordings just did not work in translation. They had to be transformed. While engaging in that, I also cut out the many footnotes to Dutch literatures and inserted others, adapted to an 'international' audience. Along the way the book gradually changed from an intervention in a Dutch public discussion, into a text that, while never denying its provincial origins, may travel widely. Or so I hope.

My greatest support in all this was John Law. He went through the manuscript several times to correct the English. And while thus doing his 'imperialist language duties', he also pointed out slippages and gaps. He encouraged me to keep on trying. And even when my work on care was still in Dutch, he attended to my stories and discussed difficult issues with me as they arose.

Many other people were helpful in those earlier stages too. I am grateful to ZON/Mw, the Netherlands Organisation for Health Research and Development, for the grant that allowed me to write this book; and to NWO, the Netherlands Organisation for Scientific Research, especially its programme 'Ethics, Research and Policy', for grants for earlier projects that leave their traces here, as well as for my current grant, that goes under the title 'Good food, good information'. The Socrates Foundation supports my one-day-a-week Socrates Chair as a Professor of Political Philosophy: I am grateful for its trust. I want to thank the philosophers in Twente, especially Hans Achterhuis, for providing me with an academic home. In hospital Z, I learned a lot, first and foremost from Edith ter Braak, Harold de Valk, Guy Rutten and Yvonne de la Bye. Claar Parlevliet and Efanne de Bok conducted good interviews and helped me to analyse them: thanks. And of course I am most grateful to all the patients who allowed me an insight into their lives with diabetes. Their identities are hidden in this book behind invented names and yet I hope that, if they come across this text, they will feel happy with the way I have used fragments of their stories.

And then I would have liked to thank Willem Erkelens, the Professor of Internal Medicine who welcomed me into his realm and encouraged me to write about what went on there, even if he regularly asked 'But when are you going to publish in a *real* journal?' – meaning a medical one. Sadly he died before this project was completed. Since this book appeared in Dutch, Lolle Nauta, exemplary intellectual and severe but supportive teacher of social philosophy, also died. As did my mother. And however much the logic of care is based on recent field work, when it comes to it, I guess, my friend Jolanda Kremer, decades ago, taught me the most about what it is to live with a disease and then to die from it.

But luckily I can still thank the people with whom I collaborated closely while we jointly and separately tried to articulate 'good care': Dick Willems, Rita Struhkamp, Tsjalling Swiertsra, and, above all, Jeannette Pols. And then there are other friends and colleagues with whom I talked about care and/or who commented on earlier versions of this text: Mieke Aerts, Marianne van den Boomen, Irene Costera Meijer, Hans Harbers, Mirjam Kohinor, Bernard Kruithof, Geertje Mak, Amâde M'charek and Nienke Uniken Venema. I also received crucial encouragement and resistance from Ingrid Baart, Conny Bellemakers, Yolan Koster-Dreese, Hilde de Jong, Brenda Diergaarde, Alice Stollmeijer, Evelien Tonkens and Pieter Pekelharing. And then there is Stefan Hirschauer to thank. He does not quite fit, for he has not yet read this text either in Dutch or in English. But the thought that he will makes me keen to be sharp.

Very early on, my father taught me what a clinical attitude entails, while my mother infused me with her geographical gaze, material and social at the same time. My current family, finally, is invaluable.

Notes

1 Two logics

1 At the end of this book you find footnotes. Most of these refer to scholarly literatures. In the genre I engage in here, literatures are not referred to in order to prove anything. Instead, they provide resonances, sidelines, points of contrast, related insights and questions. A researcher often fails to realise exactly where she draws a particular insight from; or what makes her use one term rather than another. However, it belongs to the art of academic writing to try to make (at least some of) the relations between a text and the literature explicit. Which is what I do in the footnotes. This implies that you do not need to read any footnotes in order to follow the argument of the book. However, they may help if you want to situate this argument better in the scholarly traditions that made it possible.

2 Research on other sites and situations in health care obviously informs the argument of this book in many ways. Much research has been done, and only some of it can be mentioned in the footnotes. Let me begin, however, by mentioning two studies that were crucial to my own as they were done in parallel to it. One is that of Jeannette Pols, who studied *good care* in psychiatric institutions for elderly and chronic patients. Pols focuses on something I skip over here: the relations between different *versions* of good care that clash and interfere with one another in any site and situation (Pols 2003, 2005, 2006a, 2006b). The other is that of Rita Struhkamp, who did field work in a rehabilitation centre, on wards for people with multiple sclerosis and people with spinal cord lesions (Struhkamp 2004, 2005a, 2005b). I learned a great deal from the continuous comparison between our cases.

3 The differentiation between 'individual' and 'collective' itself does not begin to make global sense. For instance, Dorinne Kondo tells that her field work in Japan calls for other categorisations (Kondo 1990). The same goes for most anthropology that takes what informants say and do not as an occasion for recognising pre-established structures but as an inspiration for novel theorising. See the exemplary work of Marilyn Strathern, who not only takes 'the others' on their own terms, but also uses these terms as theoretical tools with which to study Westerners, or, more specifically, the English (e.g. Strathern 1988 and 1992). Thus, instead of drawing images of some 'Other' so as to make the 'Western Self' come out as the better version of Man (a widespread style of reasoning that we were taught about in Saïd 1991), 'the West' itself gets objectified and opened up in novel ways.

4 Entire bookcases could be cited here. But let me restrict myself to my favourite, a book that describes the connection between the sugar cultivated by slaves in the Caribbean, and the factory workers in Britain who were fed on sweet tea. Jointly they fuelled the industrial revolution and made capitalism global from the start (see Mintz 1985; and for a follow up Mintz 1996).

5 The example comes from a book in which 'African philosophy' is analysed as 'cultural inquiry' (Shaw 2000). All philosophy pertains to specific (cultural) practices, but 'European philosophy' is all too rarely researched in this way. For some wonderful exceptions, see the essays (in Lawrence & Shapin 1998), highly relevant to the present book, that unravel how various European scientists and/or philosophers (in the seventeenth, eighteenth and nineteenth centuries) lived the daily realities of their bodies.

6 In other words, I would like to make a contribution to the task of 'provincializing Europe' (Chakrabarty 2000), by 'othering' Europe from within, using ethnographic methods. Exemplary in this respect is Bruno Latour's ethnography of a Nobel Prize-winning science laboratory for which he used the skills he had just acquired in studying school children in the Ivory Coast (Latour & Woolgar 1979). (Even if the laboratory was located in California; and the writing partly sociological.)

7 For a history of the welfare state in terms of 'chains of mutual dependency' between the inhabitants, see de Swaan 1988. For the excessive energy spent on making choices, and other disappointments implied, see Schwarz 2004. For the argument that liberalism, with its promises of choice, constrains rather than liberates those who hoped for freedom, see Santoro 2004.

8 For an original theological reflection on the empathy that may be involved in giving care to others, see Hoesset 2003. For the classic take on the gift as something that does not fit exchange, see Mauss 1990. For the argument that, just as I claim for care, the gift has not disappeared with the emergence of 'modernity' either, see Ssorin-Chaikov 2006. For the ways in which people invest care, in the form of *agapè*, in their work, see Boltanski 1990. And for the ethics of care, see the groundbreaking work of Tronto 1993; and, more recently, Hamington & Miller 2006. Of these literatures, care ethics and feminist political theory leave most traces in the present study. But while this book stands in a long feminist tradition, I will not explore the gender aspects of 'care' head-on. It is a topic that deserves separate attention. Obviously 'care' is associated with women, but that does not directly relate to the care practices examined here. Although 'the nurse' has been modelled after the housewife/mother, 'the doctor' was an incarnation of the understudied figure of the male care-giver. This figure also includes the male breadwinner, who took care of 'his' family; and the soldier who cared for his (wounded, worried) comrades. By leaving the gender of the care-giver aside to focus instead on 'care' itself, the feminism I engage in here does not seek to support 'women', but rather to interfere with the categories of our (social) understanding.

9 Over the years, many books and articles have shown that all too often in health-care practices there is just not enough kindness to go round. At the same time, 'kind' professionals find it difficult not to suffer too much along with their patients. See e.g. Hahn 1985. In his classic study of the training of surgeons, Bosk found that among these, so-called 'technical' failures may be forgiven, while 'moral' ones, i.e. not being open and decent, are not; see Bosk 1979. For

a good recent analysis as well as a plea in favour of *generosity*, that attends to the generosity of professionals as well as patients, see Frank 2004.

10 In line with the Heideggerian understanding of 'Sorge' as other to technology, writings about medical technology have mostly taken care and technology to be 'natural opposites'. The cases studied often give ample reason to stick to this approach. (See for instance Reiser 1978 and Reiser & Anbar 1984.) A different take on this has been to argue that medical technology is not opposed to, but dependent on, the hands-on work in 'the clinic'. See for this Canguilhem 1991 and 1994. In Canguilhem's approach, the practices humans engage in get precedence over whatever (representational) knowledges they may generate. As he puts it, even if a physicist could explain a disease, he would still die from it. The care articulated in the present book is a version of Canguilhem's 'clinic' (see for the difference Mol 1998; and for a related understanding, contrasting the clinic with administrative approaches, Dodier 1993 and 1998.)

11 This short paragraph opens the door to the rich academic field of disability studies. In this field 'disability' rather than 'disease' was theorised, so that studies focus on, for instance, people in wheelchairs rather than on people with cancer. (See e.g. Barnes *et al.* 2002 and Shakespeare 2006.) In line with the tradition of disability studies, the present book focuses on daily life practices of bodies-in-an-environment rather than on deviant bodies-in-isolation. However, I concentrate on care, that is on the interferences between treatment and daily life, and have little to say about equally relevant issues such as schooling, work, housing, transport facilities.

12 Present-day cognitive psychologists stress the lack of 'rationality' in the way people make choices. For an entrance into this see Schwartz 2004. The idea that ethics should attend to the conditions under which people may make choices, and thus to social issues, was interestingly put forward in the essays in Nussbaum & Sen 1993.

13 In the tradition of the nursing sciences, attempts to theorise 'care' as a multi-layered phenomenon date from long before the term was shifted into (feminist) ethics and political theory. In this context the following layers of 'caring' were separated out: caring as a human trait, a moral imperative, an affect, an interpersonal interaction and an intervention (see Morse *et al.* 1992). Approached from that tradition, the present book may prove disappointing, for it does not attend to all of these layers. Here, care is mainly studied as an intervention (or rather a style of intervening) and as an interaction (between people but also between people and materialities, i.e. technologies and bodies).

14 The philosophical discipline 'logic' seeks to formulate the rational rules of reasoning: rules for deductively drawing justified conclusions from initial premises. That I use the term in such a different way here is made easier by writings that have convincingly undermined the universalist pretensions of rationalist logic (see e.g., in feminist mode, Nye 1990.) There is also good work in anthropology that, while using the term 'logic', addresses practices (e.g. Goody 1986). This makes it easier to stretch the term for the present purposes.

15 For the term 'discourse' see e.g. Foucault 1974. In the English-language literatures, the term 'discourse' has been taken up by scholars who put it to use when analysing the languages in and of particular fields and formations. It came to resemble what might earlier have been called 'ideology' minus the Marxist overtones. (See e.g. Howarth *et al.* 2000). However, one of the more fascinating aspects of Foucault's work is that he studied language and materialities

together and, for example, wrote about cutting in corpses as a physical practice linked up with concepts such as symptom and sign, surface and depth (see Foucault 1976). John Law used the phrase 'modes of ordering' as a theoretical tool to describe a modern organisation that appeared to be ordered in various modes simultaneously; and was never finished, but always in the process of being ordered. Thus he added multiplicity as well as process, while also keeping the materialities implied in focus. See Law 1994.

16 Those who need to be convinced of the fact that 'the world' enters philosophy along with its language, would do well to read about what metaphors bring along in Lakoff & Johnson 1981. Once convinced, you may want to read the work of Michel Serres, who unravels ways in which images, structures and questions circulate through framings, words, stories and images such that philosophy will never succeed in purifying itself from 'empirical stuff' (Serres 1997 and 2007).

17 Philosophers sometimes seem to forget that not only the natural sciences, but the social sciences too, have split off from philosophy. Thus, while they tend to show respect for 'matters of fact' that fall under the jurisdiction of the natural sciences, they often carelessly dream up 'social facts' in some version of their own. As if, somehow, they are in the position to wilfully neglect all the methodological wisdom gathered in the social sciences. While there is a lot to be said for experimenting with social science methods, while attuning them better to the complexities of the world we live in (see Law 2004), this is no reason to ignore them and to freely use badly made facts as 'examples'. To do this implies that the most important rule of method is being neglected: to allow yourself to be surprised. See Stengers 1998.

18 The geographical demarcation of this study is not a constant. Different materials come from different places. I have carried out observations in only one hospital: hospital Z, a university hospital in a medium-sized town in the Netherlands. But I have talked with professionals from other hospitals and from primary care settings. Some of the people with diabetes who were interviewed come from the city in which hospital Z is situated. Others were found through personal connections of my then research assistant, Claar Parlevliet, in a small rural community situated in the central regions of the Netherlands. And then I learnt a lot from reading around. While the interviews and most websites I analysed were in Dutch, most of the social science literature that I read was 'international' – written in French or in English. At a few points in the book I will make small geographical excursions (in particular, in Chapter 5). Where I do so, this has been clearly indicated. What needs to be emphasised is that the 'Dutch' patient presented here comes with little specification. Potentially relevant differences (in age, level of education, work, literacy, original language, et cetera) are only touched upon indirectly on a few occasions. The interferences between the logic of care and the hopes, expectations and skills of different (groups of) patients, deserve further study.

19 Let me stress that the object of this study is not patients or doctors, but health-care practices – and not even 'real existing' health-care practices, but the ideals inspiring them. Thus, while I did interviews, my stories do not have the richness of the genre of the 'auto-ethnography' of people with a disability and/or a disease. See e.g. Murphy 1990; Frank 1991. I have little to say about the emotions intertwined with being a patient or with engaging in professional care

work. No doubt this is a loss, but it helped me to get a clearer insight into the practicalities of doctoring.

20 Beware: people with diabetes may have other diseases as well. Their life with diabetes is also structured by far more than their disease. Thus the 'life with diabetes' that I talk about depends on a lot of simplifications. Readers who are interested primarily in actual daily lives with diabetes would do better to read books that seek to deal with those, e.g. Roney 2000.

21 In medical sociology studying 'life with diabetes' has been linked with the study of 'modern patienthood' for many years. Claudine Herzlich and Janine Pierret already made this link in the early 1980s (see Herzlich & Pierret 1984). This was before the introduction of the miniature blood sugar monitor that is so relevant to current diabetes self-care. In their broad historical perspective, Herzlich and Pierret contrast diabetes with the epidemic diseases of old, which caused fever, were infectious, attacked large anonymous groups of people at the same time, and required social measures from above. One of the many interesting differences with that older 'regime' that Herzlich and Pierret point to, is that in diabetes the person who is being taken care of also, always and necessarily takes care of herself. This, along with a positive identification with fellow sufferers in patient groups, or so they claim, marks 'modern patients'. At about the same time other sociologists, signalling how much patients (and the people close to them) have to *do*, started to talk about these activities as *work*. See Strauss *et al.* 1985.

22 See Bliss 1982 for the history of the isolation of insulin and the early experiments with injecting it from the outside. For a history of what thus became of living with the disease, see Freudtner 2003.

2 Customer or patient?

1 Of course, markets also come in different shapes and sizes. The (simplified!) market I refer to here is the one that is both articulated and co-shaped by neo-classical economic theory. For a sociology of the market that does not take neo-classical economy to describe its object, but rather to inform it, see Callon 1998. The introduction of market language, meanwhile, is not the only form of 'economisation' possible. There are several others, such as the ideal of working efficiently, which have slightly different connotations. See Ashmore *et al.* 1989.

2 In my field, mmol/l was the commonly used unit for the concentration of blood sugar and this is the custom I follow in this book. Elsewhere mg/dL is in use. If you have trouble making a quick calculation from one unit to the other, then imagine what happens if you have diabetes and travel from a country with one tradition to one with the other. This is made even more difficult since not only blood sugar levels but also units of insulin are not expressed in a universal way: standards differ between countries.

3 Obviously money is a crucial element in health-care practices. It is quite an intervention to bracket it off. This is one more simplification that must help to tease out the logic of care that is so difficult to disentangle from complex practices. How it might be drawn in again, without reductively claiming that, when it comes to it, everything comes down to money, is a challenging task. For an interesting attempt to analyse how people working in the pharmaceutical industry deal with money as well as morality, see Martin 2006.

4 As customers, our position in capitalism seems to be far better than as workers.

For workers do not own the means of production they work with, but customers çan choose and thus believe that they are in charge. This feeds into a profound shift in Western countries: worker identities have made place for customer identities. See Lury 1996.

5 That products which change hands on markets have a beginning and an end and may be isolated from their surroundings is not a natural feature of the objects involved. It is an effect of how they are shaped. Various studies that go back to earlier phases of capitalism reveal the effort that this took. See the essays in Appadurai 1986 and Thomas 1991. In the light of this work, it would be naïve to say that it is *impossible* to turn health care into a market. It can be done. But, and this is what I do argue, a lot would be lost along the way. (Which begs the question as to whether it might also be possible to (still, again) think of interesting alternatives for the existing markets for (other) 'goods' – but this is beyond the scope of the present study.) In many places, for instance in the North American context, marketisation has gone a lot further than in the Netherlands. Various North American authors seek to spell out what indeed they are losing in the process (see e.g. Callahan & Wasunna 2006). This may make Dutch field work all the more relevant and interesting!

6 The conference 'Customers in Careland' was organised by the branch of ZON/Mw (the Dutch organisation for health-care research) that also provided financial support for the present project. I was a speaker at this conference too, invited to explain in one of the parallel workshop sessions why patients might perhaps *not* benefit from being called 'customers in careland'. Some people in the audience responded to my talk with relief – finally someone who voiced what they had already been thinking. Others, however, were actively engaged in (often good) initiatives that went under headings like 'customer-oriented care'. They were annoyed by what they took to be my 'scepticism'. Why did I not want to improve the position of 'customers'? Such things happen when one engages in theoretical reflection in a practically oriented environment, where terms are not so much discussed but used to the best of people's abilities.

7 Some people who read earlier versions of this text urged me to take out this reference to my being ill. As it happened, I was ill for much of the time that I was working on this book, but why was this relevant to the reader? Or, another concern, why would I make myself vulnerable by mentioning it? As you can see, I did not take it out. First, as to making myself vulnerable: we *are* vulnerable, all of us, and since one of the aims of this book is to underline this, I can use this as an occasion for doing so. Second, of course the state of health of an author is not particularly relevant to a reader. What counts is whether or not the resulting text is interesting. But then again: the particularities of researchers interfere with their work. If I had been more ill than I was, I would not have been able to do research and to write at all. But at the same time, my illness might well have increased my sensitivity to presumptions of unmarked normality. Academia tends to take the 'health' of scholars for granted: it usually goes unanalysed. For an interesting exception, see Golledge 1997, where the author makes explicit what he had to change in his professional practices as an academic geographer when, later in life, he became blind. In the present book I have not seriously analysed the interferences between my personal particularities and my work, but make use of my passion for walking as well as the instructiveness of *not* fitting in with other people's expectations ('you and me'), as incidental reminders that knowledge and theorising are always situated. For questions to

do with the intersection of 'auto' and 'ethnography' see also e.g. Okely & Call-away 1992, who talk of autobiography; and Menely & Young 2005, who take the 'auto' they reflect on not as private, but as academic life.

8   The ways in which patients were gradually turned into members of the care team in the course of the second half of the twentieth century has for some while been noted and sceptically explored by a small number of sociologists of medicine. In their writing they took this as a form of medicalising that tended to silence possible patient resistance to medical power. The patient-subject that they saw being created is a mixture of the subject of choice and the subject of care that I am carefully trying to differentiate in the present book. For two dif-ferent but equally compelling studies, see Armstrong 1983 and Arney & Bergen 1984. Both books are very good antidotes to the belief that patients gain 'freedom' as they become addressed as subjects of care and/or choice. However, since these books suggest that what goes on is, instead, a form of sub-mission, they are still caught in the autonomy–heteronomy dichotomy that I am trying to escape from here.

9   'Walking itself' is obviously not a natural, a-historical category but a recent, and culturally highly specific, invention. See for this Solnit 2006.

10 How could one tell who is the patient and who is not in an advertisement? First, diabetes is not visible. And second, this image, or so my informant told me, may well have targeted the Dutch market, but came from an American agency that specialises in making and selling photographs for advertising. It is highly unlikely that the agency asks models about their medical condition, so they may have all kinds of diseases, or none at all. Potential buyers of a blood sugar monitor, then, are seduced into buying a product by models who look vital and are probably healthy as well. This is quite like the way 17-year-old girls are used to show that, 'thanks to our wonderful product', it is possible to keep a smooth and youthful skin. For this, and more generally for learning to 'read' adverts, see Coward 1996.

11 For the term absence/presence, see Law 2002. Law shows how much of what is involved in shaping a technology is not necessarily immediately visible in the here and now. He traces the design of a warplane and the ways in which factors like the enemy Russians; the flying distance to base camps; pilots' tendency to get sick if movements are too violent; and a lot more, are all 'present' in the design even if only in indirect ways. At the first level they are absent.

12 That 'no' is impossible to sell, makes it absurd to think that organising health care as a market might make things cheaper than alternative organisational forms, especially those that organise care in such a way that 'needs' are being addressed while limits to what can be done are respected. Along with the market, a 'regime of hope' is rapidly expanding in health care; fed by research practices partially embedded in industry and privately funded, which promise return-on-investment, financially as well as in terms of 'health gain'. See Moreira & Palladino 2005. For further analysis, and an attempts to frame the 'sociology of expectations' appropriate to the analysis of what is going on here, see Brown & Michael 2003.

13 Non-heroic care comes with patient narratives in which living with a disease is also no longer told as a heroic endeavour in which a disease-enemy is to be harshly fought and conquered so as to avoid sliding into fatalism. For an inter-

esting analysis of alternative possibilities, see Diedrich 2005; and for one of the narratives that she reflects upon, Stacey 1997.

3 The citizen and the body

1 In this chapter I consider theories that define the citizen. For an example of a study that follows how patient laws work in practice, see Jeannette Pols's comparison between two psychiatric wards: one where the professionals followed the letter of the law and another where they didn't. In the first people were respected as free citizens up until a pivotal moment, when, with all the forms signed, they might be put into (temporary) seclusion. In the latter professionals openly admitted that they manipulate people. But they never locked anyone up, however wild with madness they might be. To do so would spoil their relations with them; see Pols 2003. My approach makes less difference *inside* health care, but tries to learn *from* health care. It is interesting to note that some of the most creative 'general' social theory in the twentieth century resulted from studies that took health care as their exemplary domain. See, most notably, Parsons 1951 and Foucault 1967.

2 Despite the theoretical clash between emancipation and feminism as political strategies, in practical political situations these approaches have often strengthened rather than undermined each other. For the Netherlands this has been beautifully analysed in Aerts 1991; but the phenomenon is not exclusively Dutch (see also Scott 1999). That the content of the categories 'women' and 'men' is not stable but may alter, and alter fast, was nicely shown in Costera Meijer 1991. It is interesting to note here that, while 'constructivism' and 'feminism' had tense relations in many places, in the Netherlands they have been thought together since the early 1980s. See also Hirschauer & Mol 1995. This may have helped me in framing 'patientism'. For the interference between differences between the sexes and differences between 'healthy' and 'unhealthy' people, see Moser 2006.

3 Talking about health as the 'silence of the organs' is a reference to Canguilhem who says he took it from Lerich. It suggests that health is something we are unaware of. Disease, by introducing chaos/noise, attracts our attention. But, says Canguilhem, disease is not chaos. An organism only stays alive as long as it is able to re-establish some alternative order. See Canguilhem 1991. The image comes back in the work of Michel Serres when he argues that there is no such thing as cleanliness or pure order, because all attempts at ordering include a 'parasite' (one form of noise or another) just as bodies always live with parasites, too. See Serres 2007.

4 A lot of (neo-liberal) theorising about medicine models the relation between professionals and patients not just after that of feudal lords and serfs, but also, in quasi-Marxist mode, of that between ruling class and proletariat: they are in permanent opposition to one another. Real Marxists have always warned against this: they sought to analyse the relations between professionals and lay people as either strengthening or undermining class struggle. For a great article that succeeded in actually doing this, differentiating between doctors supporting miners and doctors supporting mining companies, each holding on to a different definition of 'black lung disease', see Smith 1981. Here I do not analyse 'tensions between classes (of people)' but 'tensions between logics'. How these might

interfere with one another is yet another question that I leave out of the present analysis.

5 The analysis of the Greek citizen-actor and his body that I present here comes from Kuriyama 1999, a truly wonderful book. It makes a comparison between Chinese and Greek medicine using the contrast to gain insight into both. Here I only mobilise Kuriyma's suggestion that the concept of muscle and that of an autonomous will are linked up. This muscular notion of autonomy has survived in political theory. Current 'medicine' also deals with muscles, but it is such a heterogeneous conglomerate of practices and insights, that I dare to contrast the muscular Greek citizen with the metabolic actors relevant to diabetes care. Kuriyama makes a different kind of contrast. He talks about Chinese doctors, who did not see muscles, but (when feeling the pulse) sensed *mo*. Sensing *mo*, facilitating the flow of *chi* or *xi*, and many other possibilities of living as and with bodies, are unanalysed in the present study. In its specificities, the logic of care that I try to articulate here, is provincial. It comes from a small province of the West.

6 While people with bulimia or anorexia, who are constantly preoccupied with their food, are treated for being neurotic, an all but neurotic preoccupation with food is imposed on people with diabetes. And while dieticians tend to advise people who are too fat to throw out their scales, people with diabetes are encouraged always to count their carbohydrate intake and measure their blood sugars. Such striking differences between adjacent practices are understudied. See also Cohn 1997 about diabetes and diets.

7 See James 1999 for a detailed and subtle elaboration of the various understandings of passions within political theory.

8 The history of manners has been described in Elias 2000. He points out that, if etiquette books warn against certain 'bad manners', these were apparently commonly engaged in. Foucault later addressed the disciplining of bodies of soldiers who were drilled in order to become one fighting body; and that of schoolchildren who were seated straight, in rows in classrooms. These practices turned them into the disciplined citizens who populate Foucault's political theory. See Foucault 1991.

9 Foucault's analyses have made 'normalising' sound harsh to us, while 'nourishing' sounds a lot more friendly. It might be interesting to try to abstain from an immediate judgemental reflex in both cases, and instead to explore what is being done, by whom, for whom, in which ways and to what effects. In his later work, Foucault also shifted to doing this, as when he analysed older traditions of the 'care for the self' (Foucault 1990). The relevant ideals of care articulated there have left traces in later caring practices for selves as well as for others. This suggests that professional care is secondary to self-care. This also emerges from, for instance, studies of the medical work of Descartes, who did not require an intermediary (i.e. a professional doctor) between medical science and its application but applied his own science to himself and advised his friends to do likewise (Shapin 2000).

10 The dream of escaping from the body infuses large parts of philosophy. And yet bodies have been reflected on in the philosophical tradition in a variety of ways. See for instance Vallega-Neu 2005; or, focusing on bodily metaphors in philosophy, Lakoff & Johnson 1999. Some even argue that Kant, so easily cast here (as elsewhere) as requiring us to escape from our bodies in order to think critically, can be read in an entirely different way, i.e. as someone exploring the philosophical implications of human embodiment (Svare 2006).

11 In the history of medicine and biology, this deterministic, causal way of understanding bodies is not very old. It emerged along with laboratory research in the
nineteenth century. For an interesting history of its emergence that situates it
among its alternatives, see Pickstone 2000.

12 Thus, my point here is not, like that of phenomenology, that next to the body
that we 'have' (which is known from the outside), we should also pay attention
to the body we 'are' (experienced from the inside). I make a different claim
which is that in the clinic the most relevant body is the body we 'do'. It is a part
of practices. For more extensive versions of this argument, see Mol 2002a and b
and Mol & Law 2004. For the argument that anthropologists studying 'the
body' should not accept its dominant definitions, but seek to redefine their
object, see Taylor 2005. Meanwhile the most detailed and gripping study of
what may become of bodies in care practices that I know of is that of the
'Research centre for shared incompetence' Xperiment! This group has assembled images of care work, showing bodies caring as well as bodies cared-for, in a
clinic for people who cannot actively move their own bodies. These were presented on a 320 m² display in the exhibition 'Making Things Public' at the ZKM
in Karlsruhe in 2005. For a trace of this, see Xperiment! 2005.

13 Alertness and aliveness are needed for the use of technologies in other diseases
too. See, for the case of performing dialysis at home, Wen-yuan Lin 2005; for
living with inhalers and peak flow meters, Willems 1998; for dealing with one's
wheelchair, Winance 2006. Willems argues that the ability to care for themselves with technologies provides patients with *agency* rather than *autonomy*
(Willems 2002). This is what, in a slightly different way, I also try to argue
here.

14 That the body is not a 'naturally given' phenomenon becomes interestingly clear
when its abilities to sense – to see, hear, feel, smell, taste – are attended to.
These are far from universal. They have a history and differ between cultures.
For an overview, see Classen 1993. In specific historical and cultural sites their
shaping is not necessarily widely shared either, but depends on practices. Thus,
'a person' may gradually become 'an amateur of music', through practices of
listening and learning to differentiate sounds (see Hennion 2001). Others learn
to distinguish between wines while simultaneously acquiring an extensive
vocabulary that allows for subtle differentiations that the non-initiated simply
cannot taste (see Teil 2004). A body, or so Hennion and Teil tell us, does not
passively experience what is 'out there', but gradually 'learns to be affected'.
For a classic version of this argument in sociology, see Becker 1953.

15 The senses and technologies each have their own diagnostic strengths. Thus:
diagnosing anaemia with an Hb-measurement device is the 'gold standard' and
the 'more accurate' approach, but diagnosing by lowering an eyelid and assessing its colour requires less time, fewer tools and technicians, is less risky, and
accurate enough to 'catch' cases of severe anaemia. All in all it *transports* better
to far-away places (see Mol & Law 1994). Or: in the course of brain surgery,
the apparatus of the anaesthetists and the fingers of the surgeon may come to
different conclusions about the patient's blood pressure. And yet in practice
neither is trusted alone at the expense of the other: they are used interdepen-
dently (see Moreira 2006).

16 There are exceptions. Sometimes medical advice is legally binding. For
instance, as I just mentioned, in many countries the law requires doctors to state
whether or not their patients with diabetes are capable of driving a car or not.

Many doctors dislike this since it runs counter to the logic of care. However, it is also rarely mentioned in discussions about patient choice, as it also seems to go against the logic of choice because doctors rather than patients suddenly have to make the decisions. However, liberalism would be able to defend itself here because a patient who unwisely chose to drive would pose a danger to other road users. Meanwhile, the examples that *are* used in discussions about patient choice, tend to take one side immediately with 'patient choice': cases of arrogant abuse of professional power are easy to find. (At the extreme end, there are always the Nazi doctors to remember; see e.g. Lifton 1988.) One of the tasks that comes with 'not frustrating emancipation but going beyond it' is to find ways of tackling abuses of power with suitable, but not necessarily neo-liberal, repertoires.

4 Managing versus doctoring

1 That I was even able to *see* that in clinical practice knowledge and technology work in ways very different from how they tend to be presented is due to a large number of studies that have gradually built the alternative image I sketch below. These studies have a mixed background. For one, in the early 1980s the history of medicine made a radical shift. Instead of describing emerging knowledge as a matter of 'facts discovered', it began to talk about its 'construction'. See for this early work Wright & Treacher 1982. At the same time medical anthropologists no longer restricted their studies to 'healers' in non-Western cultures, but started to do field work in Western hospitals, in part to help professionals understand their 'strange' patients (see e.g. Kleinman 1980). However, once they started to do this, they also began to study professionals – an intriguing 'culture' in its own right (see e.g. Stein 1990). There was an overlap with sociologists, some of whom also did field work, that gradually shifted its attention from (power) relations between people, to the content of what was being done (see e.g. Prior 1989). Meanwhile, 'science and technology studies' emerged. In this field scholars studied laboratories and other sites and situations where scientific papers were written, technological tools developed and new materials were put together (see Latour & Woolgar 1979). In the 1990s, these various types of inquiry began to encounter each other and to cross over. See e.g. Epstein 1996; Berg 1997; Berg & Mol 1998; Lock *et al.* 2000.

2 The term 'normative fact' comes from the medical literature. I first encountered it when investigating how 'normal Hb' gets established, where Hb stands for 'haemoglobin level' and 'normal Hb' is used as a standard for assessing the presence or absence of anaemia. In some of the articles we analysed for that study, a 'normal Hb' was explicitly called a 'normative fact'. While philosophers often took great pains to distinguish norms from facts, I was immediately taken by the term (see Mol & Berg 1994). Be warned that, even if my analysis complexifies 'normative facts', what I am writing here is still a simplification. It leaves out such things as differences between the standards set by different laboratories; inaccuracies of the measurements involved; shifting accuracies of various machines; the consequences of using mmol/l rather then mg/dL as a unit; and so on.

3 Van Haeften 1995: p. 142, original in Dutch.

4 Ter Braak 2000: p. 188, original in English.

5 A lot of diagnostic techniques are not even put to use if there is no promise of a

therapeutic intervention on the horizon; and the ways in which they are being used depends on the treatment options under consideration. See for this Mol & Elsman 1996. In the course of a procedure such as performing an operation, the questions of what to do and what the matter is may also keep on informing each other in a process of shaping and reshaping what exactly is being done (see Moreira 2006).

6 Rita Struhkamp offers a far more detailed analysis of setting and shifting treatment goals in rehabilitation practice. She argues that it makes eminent sense to set goals because this gives therapy some sort of orientation. But along the way things tend to shift, because bodies prove more or less difficult than expected and a person's wishes and priorities gradually take different forms. But if goals are set to have something tangible to tinker with, something goes wrong if they are simultaneously being used to evaluate treatment. Instead, it would be better to design evaluations that take into account that in the course of therapy the goals are fluid and adaptable. See Struhkamp 2004.

7 Arguing against squeezing technology into means–end distinctions, Bruno Latour has proposed that we face what he so eloquently calls *the end of the means*. And so we should. See Latour 2002.

8 The question of the strengths and limits of the RCT, the Randomized Clinical Trial, as a research strategy, is too large to take on here. It is, however, relevant for my argument. Take the requirement of the RCT method to pick the parameters for success early on. This not only blocks insight into the unexpected, but means that the parameters may not be neutral between the treatments being compared. For instance, in many trials of rehabilitation techniques, 'muscle strength' was used as a parameter while one of the interventions assessed was primarily about preventing muscle spasms (see Lettinga & Mol 1999). What exactly to compare with what is not always obvious: thus for walking therapy to succeed, 'talking' is essential, while surgeons who operate do not take it to be a part of treatment, but 'mere social glue' (see Mol 2002b). The requirement of a so-called 'control group' and of 'double blinds' may also have unintended effects (see Dehue 2005). Trials moreover only test what has been developed elsewhere, and they are not innovative in and of themselves. What is more: because so much money is at stake, and trials are so decisive, they are often used to push drugs through rather than to test them (see Healy 2004), while the practice of the trial itself may be as much a marketing tool as research (see Pignarre 1997).

9 It often happens that new diagnostic techniques, or new possibilities for intervention, change the definition of the diseases they sought to diagnose or intervene in (see e.g. Pasveer 1992). More generally: what a disease *is* in the practices of diagnosing and treating it, depends on the technologies with which it is being diagnosed and treated. This, then, implies that diseases are far from single coherent entities. There are many diagnostic and therapeutic technologies, and each technology enacts a slightly different version of the object it interferes with. This in turn implies that one of the more impressive tasks hospitals (researchers, clinicians, patients) face is to coordinate the varied versions of any 'one disease' in such a way that it does not fall apart. See for this Mol 2002a and b.

10 What at first sight looks like 'the same' technique or technology may work in quite different ways depending on context and use. In their detailed comparisons of different practices of giving birth, Madeleine Akrich and Bernike

Pasveer show that similarities and differences may be layered upon each other in quite complex ways. They also note that 'the body itself', is not a natural phenomenon, but differs between birth settings with the technologies used, and over the course of giving birth. See Akrich & Pasveer 2000 and 2004.

11 While the logic of care may want technologies to be adaptable and fluid, they are not necessarily like this. Some technologies are made in ways that allow for more adaptability than others. In health care, it is often (though not necessarily always) the case that laboratory techniques require more procedural and material consistency than clinical techniques, which may be more easily adapted by the skilful professionals who mobilise them (see Mol & Law 1994). However, even if technologies look remarkably solid and sturdy, they may be built in such a way that they are adaptable and able to accommodate change – or not. Since all technologies are likely to fail sooner or later, adaptability and reparability might well be listed among the more important requirements of 'good technology'. For this argument, see de Laet & Mol 2000.

12 For a version of the argument that expertise should be brought under democratic control, see Rip *et al.* 1995. In the context of health care the question has been raised time and time again as to what extent professionals can and should control each other, and to what extent they should be controlled from the outside (see e.g. Freidson 2001). One of the arguments for 'self-control' is that professions have access to a large body of specialised knowledge and that working with medical technologies requires specialised skills. If, however, the very heart of professional work, the *doctoring*, is being turned into teamwork, then it makes sense to suggest that 'self-control' should be teamwork too. Not something that happens inside, nor something from the outside, but something that involves the blurring and shifting of boundaries.

5 Individual and collective

1 The genetic image of genes that move from one generation to the next has absorbed older images of the 'inheritance' of money and other possessions. See, for an analysis of this in the British context, Strathern 1992. Other old images also surface in popular parlance about 'genes' and 'offspring' in a fairly direct manner – often interfering in unexpected ways with the latest attempts of 'science' to alter them. For a German example, see Duden 2002. For more enquiries into genetic (self-)understandings and practices, see Goodman *et al.* 2003.

2 For an analysis of variously framed 'individuals' that figure within social theory, see Michael 2006. For an impressive historical analysis of various framings of the individual in twentieth-century health care, see Armstrong 2002.

3 Proponents of patient choice often suggest that it is easier (nicer, less humiliating) to depend on technologies than to depend on other people. In practice, this isn't necessarily the case. For some counter-stories, see Struhkamp 2004. Meanwhile, it is not only patients who owe their ability to act to others. This goes for all of us. Interestingly, this has been wonderfully shown for the case of those audacious medical professionals, who embody the image of masterful actorship *par excellence*: surgeons. See Hirschauer 1994 and Moreira 2004.

4 A group of Inuit commissioned an anthropologist to unravel the details of their high incidence of diabetes for them (see Rock 2003). See also Rock 2005, for a wider anthropological analysis of the issue of genes and environment in the case

of diabetes. Thanks to Melanie Rock for drawing my attention to the issue and for sending me her articles. I made extensive use of them in writing this chapter.

5 In broad strokes, I sketch three different concepts of 'population' here. This will do to illustrate my point. But there are further 'population' concepts around. When unravelling a court case where the suspect happened to be 'Turkish' – but what *is* 'Turkish'? – Amâde M'charek found that no less than six different concepts of 'population' were used in alternation in the course of discussion – each with a different version on what it is to be 'Turkish'. See M'charek 2005.

6 In Europe, we tend to avoid the term 'race'. In the United States it is common. American anti-racists do not avoid the term but try to give it a sociological turn. They argue that the poor health of Afro-Americans is related to their social position rather than to the colour of their skin, and that 'race' is therefore not a biological but a social category (see e.g. LaVeist 2002). And yet, in all talk of races and genes, the shadow of *eugenics* looms. It has been too powerful in the twentieth century for it to be safely neglected (see Duster 2003). To be reminded that racist modes of thinking and acting may stubbornly live on, whether or not the *term* 'race' is actually used, read the essays in Brah & Coombes 2000. But then, blocking the body out of social theory altogether is not productive either. The better strategy seems to not forget about, but to rethink the body. See e.g. Haraway 1997 and Mol 1991.

7 Genetic research does not treat us all equally, but differences other than those to do with genes are also relevant to its practices. For instance, the practicalities of acquiring DNA material are crucial to the issue of *whose* DNA got mapped when 'the human genome' was investigated. See for this again M'charek 2005. At the moment, research gets to be done more and more on populations that are easy to research. These appear to be poor people in countries that are poor, but rich enough that there are ambitious researchers and doctors around who can do part of the research. This is why a French company tried to test its drugs against bipolar disorder in Argentina rather than in France (see Lakoff 2006). At the same time, regions or neighbourhoods in India where industrial plants have just closed down are being turned into test sites because so-called 'volunteers' for clinical studies are so easy to find in such locations. For this, and more generally for a striking analysis of the way venture capitalism and biotechnology are currently jointly shaping 'biocapitalism', see Sunder Rajan 2006.

8 One of the many problems with food is that cheap food has more calories (in the form of sugar and fat) and less vitamins and proteins than expensive food. In many countries, moreover, the ties between industry and advisory bodies are so tight, that public policy does not disentangle itself sufficiently from industrial interests. For this argument, see Nestle 2002; for a wider range of cultural food issues, see Watson & Caldwell 2005. While nutrigenomics gives rise to discussions about whether the effects of food on health should either be understood in genetic or in cultural terms, our best bet may well be to become much more sophisticated about the ways in which they interact. For an inspiring example, see Nabhan 2006.

9 Thanks to Ariane de Ranitz, who, as a medical student, examined this material for me.

10 For the way public health came to be structured around the microbe, see Latour 1988. Intertwined with public health efforts, a specific way for delineating and

calculating 'populations' was established: that of statistics. In the nineteenth century statistics came to inform many emerging fields, and not least public health. It not only created 'the probable' – as a new figure between the known and the unknown – but also offered a quite specific take on people. In statistical calculations 'people' are turned into separate 'variables'. These isolated characteristics are subsequently what counts and what is counted with. See Hacking 1990 and Gigerenzer *et al.* 1989.

11 In the 1960s the large amount of people who needed care but did not come and ask for it was deemed to be a huge problem. The term 'iceberg phenomenon' was coined. Just like people in ships only see the top of an iceberg, while the rest stays below the water, so doctors only see the few patients who present themselves, while the rest stay out of their field of vision. There are still a lot of 'brave people', but these days the worry has shifted to what is called 'overconsumption'. It is interesting that Lies Henstra, who happens to have little formal education, is still able to remark on the iceberg phenomena with admirable lucidity.

6 The good in practice

1 Medical ethics started out at least in part because the image of the powerful doctor, deciding about life and death, offered a great example of a 'moral actor' whose ethical considerations were fascinating to think with. For this argument, see Toulmin 1998. The idea only gradually developed that, if there were crucial decisions to be taken, the patient was, or should be, the relevant moral actor. Social scientists, meanwhile, have had a complicated relation with medical ethics from its earliest phases. A lot of the normative issues that they, too, believed to be important, were taken up by ethics but in an entirely different way: individual actors were treated as decisive in the absence of much attention to 'contexts'. At the same time ethics was much more successful in attracting wide social attention (see e.g. Weisz 1990). The question as to whether to compete with ethics about how to frame moral issues, or whether to study 'ethics practices' as an object in its own right as one of the elements of the current medical domain, continues to present itself as a matter of urgency. For an interesting example of the latter strategy, see Hoeyer 2006.

2 Thus I do not argue for the kind of 'ethics of care' that would give care-specific answers to the so called 'unavoidable ethical questions' that arise if we have to give *reasons* for our actions. In care, the good and the bad are not in the reasons, but in the *doing* itself. For this argument, see also Harbers *et al.* 2002, which talked about a crisis in a nursing home that faced the problem of demented people refusing food. While the doctors saw this refusal as a symptom of dementia, various ethicists argued in Dutch newspapers that the people concerned were expressing their 'will to die' non-verbally by refusing food. In day-to-day life on the ward, meanwhile, neither 'nature' and its 'causes' nor the 'will' and its 'reasons' were of much importance. Instead, nurses and care assistants, without many words, tried in practical ways to make eating attractive. They mashed or didn't mash food, engaged in spoon-feeding, or provided people with food that tasted of chocolate. They tried to give *good care*.

3 In medical sociology and medical anthropology much has been written about the stories people tell about disease, care and their own lives. It has been emphasised that telling such stories is not only a way of representing reality, but may

also have therapeutic effects. For a sociological take on this see Frank 1995 and Burry 2001; and for the argument that patient narratives should have a more prominent place inside medicine, Greenhalgh & Hurwitz 1998.

4   See for this history, Bliss 1982.

5   What might be suitable terms for talking about physical collectivity? The term 'biological citizenship', coined by Adriana Petryna in her analysis of the aftermath of the accident at the nuclear power plant in Cherñobyl, does not work well, since it is meant to do something very different. Petryna's concern is with claims citizens may have on the state due to their 'biology' (Petryna 2002). Here, however, my point is not about the claims that people make, but rather about the activities that they actively engage in as they try to help. Those activities cannot be caught by that other famous term, 'biopolitics', either (see e.g. Rabinow & Rose 2006). For while 'biopolitics' seeks to encompass everything that individuals might do 'in the name of individual and collective health', the term evokes a strategy that comes from elsewhere, and a power that subjects us as it turns us into subjects. In contrast with this, in articulating the logic of care, I have sought terms that do not presume us to be either free or subjected, or both, but rather terms that try to avoid this dichotomy.

6   The doctor-with-a-disease is an interesting figure when one wants to think about the 'active patient'. He or she, after all, is officially both a scientific expert and a suffering body. See e.g. the beautiful analysis in Sacks 1984. For the many shifts involved when doctors become patients, see also Ingstad & Christie 2001. And for a truly impressive 'patient narrative' of someone who is also an expert on the body, see the article of the biologist of autopoiesis Varela about life after a liver transplant (Varela 2001).

7   That 'making decisions' is not necessarily an attractive kind of activity becomes most clear when one encounters people who try to avoid it. For an insightful and moving example of this, see Callon & Rabeharisoa 2004.

8   Studies that concentrate on what actors actually 'do' show that even 'doing nothing' is far from easy. It requires hard work. See for this the analysis that Stefan Hirschauer made of people who, when they meet in a confined space such as a lift, do a lot in order to do nothing, and especially to not 'meet' (Hirschauer 2005). And even suffering involves activity: physical pain is not something people undergo, but something they actively negotiate and tinker with. Thus, Rita Struhkamp found that people may accept days of pain and misery as a 'price to pay' for a special event, like a wedding, that they are particularly eager to attend. And 'undergoing pain', too, comes in different varieties: one may try to fight back, or try to let go, struggle or surrender. See Struhkamp 2005b.

9   Like the more neutral notion of 'experience', 'enjoyment' and 'pleasure' are not naturally occurring events either. They require effort and need to be learned. This topic is explored in an article that talks about, and compares, the 'active surrender' of amateurs of classical music and hard drug users. However different in many respects, they appear to prepare in similar ways in order to be open and receptive. They actively engage in their passion. See Gomart & Hennion 1999.

10   Obviously patients can also contribute to research on their disease in various ways. There are a range of possible roles for this, e.g. those of co-decision-maker, knowledge-bearer and/or that of someone who experiments with (his/her own) treatment. Early experience with patients in active roles in

research was acquired in the context of HIV/AIDS. For the United States this has been well documented and analysed in Epstein 1996; for France, see Bardbot 2002 and Dodier 2003. Also fascinating in this context is the French organisation for patients with muscular dystrophy, that went so far as to hire its own sociologists to study and enrich its strategies (see Rabeharisoa & Callon 1999).

11 For this history, see Marks 1997. In my attempt to show the limits of this method, I here assume that it works well for what it claims to do, but not for a lot of other things. However, when one looks at this more carefully, this assumption crumbles. So much money is involved that it is no wonder that a method that has been used for so long is also being misused in many ways. See e.g. Pignarre 1997; Healy 2004.

12 The question as to how to incorporate what is important to technology users in technologies, has been extensively studied. The first step was to uncover the 'inbuilt user' incorporated in technologies (see Woolgar 1991). A second step was to analyse variants in this user (see e.g. Oudshoorn & Pinch 2005). At the same time the issue arose as to how the 'inbuilt user' might be changed. One of the models for this is to call for a democratic gathering where designs of technologies are discussed and decided upon. Another is that of the experiment: in this, new technologies are introduced on a small scale, so that their various expected and unexpected effects can be explored. Since clinical trials that study the effectiveness and effectivity of interventions can only deal with expected effects, other, qualitative, research methods are required. See for this De Vries & Horstman 2007.

13 A remarkable example is Julian Tudor Hart's analysis of what does not work in present-day British health care. This is a critical book, but its criticism is not directed at professionals but at the conditions under which they are made to work. These limit clinical ways of working – or what in the present study I have called doctoring. Care (Tudor Hart 2006).

14 Michel Foucault suggested the term 'heterotopia' as an alternative to that other elsewhere, the 'utopia', which is a good place that one may dream about, an idealisation (Foucault 1986). A heterotopia not only fosters other values, but also holds other styles of evaluation than the topos one starts out from. Foucault advised us to look for heterotopias as vantage points from which to study the place in which we find ourselves. Just as history allows us to cast new light on the present, heterotopias make it possible to better understand, say, the West. In anthropology this has been amply experimented with. I already mentioned the work of Marilyn Strathern (e.g. Strathern 1992). In philosophy the most fascinating attempt in this direction that I know of is the work of François Julien, who reads Chinese philosophy as a heterotopic elsewhere that allows him to reinterpret Greek philosophy in highly original ways (Julien 2000). While the scholarly unravelling of classic Chinese thought and field work articulating present-day daily life with diabetes in the Netherlands are obviously very different from each other in ever so many ways, as modes of interfering with philosophy they are related.

15 Of course numerous 'logics' *are* being unravelled. An interesting example, with resonances to the logic of care, is the recent work of Donna Haraway, in which she seeks to articulate the specificities of the relations between humans and dogs in terms of companionship (Haraway 2003). For an attempt to develop the notion of non-human friendship, even with animals who are not quite companions, see Bingham 2006.

16   The idea of the West as a complex composition circulates in many versions in social theorising. See Law 1994, who presents *modes of ordering* as co-existing, clashing and interfering while they jointly shape a 'modern organization'. Or see Thévenot 2006, who proposes that we study 'régimes d'engagement' (and shows a way to do so). For an excerpt of this in English, see Thévenot 2002.

17   That they may mix, is one of the more striking differences between the 'logics' I try to present here, and the 'spheres of justice' that are presented in Walzer 1983. Spheres of justice, like regions, are adjacent to one another. Logics may interfere. The fact that they may do so, is linked up with their being embedded in practices. In her wonderful book about English and Yoruba systems of counting, Helen Verran has shown that, when we approach these as two ways of *thinking*, they inevitably clash, so that the question as to which of them is better can only be avoided by relativism. However, if we approach them as a way of *practising* counting, a lot of interferences, divisions of labour, cross-overs and other combinations become possible. Thus we may yet live together (Verran 2001).

18   Ecology and ecological problems seem an obvious terrain where some variant of the logic of care might be of immediate relevance. See for this e.g. Hinchliffe 2007. The point is neither to celebrate warm motherly care at the cost of a more political approach, nor to turn against technology, but to reframe what politics and what technology themselves entail. See Latour & Weibel 2005; and Barry 2001.

19   Interesting in this context are attempts to theorise the practice of 'engaging in research', as if it were, or should be, a caring practice. This might imply that instead of seeking to establish 'matters of fact', research should address 'matters of concern' (Latour 2004). This resonates with a much older hope of the Starnberger study group that clinical research might set a good example for the natural sciences. Just as medicine is oriented towards 'health', the natural sciences, they said, were in need of explicit normative goals, too (Böhme *et al.* 1978). In this context it is also interesting to recall Bruno Latour's plea for framing our relation to technology in terms of *love* (Latour 1997).

Literature

Aerts, M. (1991) Just the Same or Just Different? a Feminist Dilemma, in J. Hermsen & A. van Lenning, eds, *Sharing the Difference: Feminist Debates in Holland*, London: Routledge, pp. 23–31

Akrich, M. & B. Pasveer (2000) Multiplying Obstetrics: Techniques of Surveillance and Forms of Coordination, *Theoretical Medicine and Bioethics*, vol. 21, 63–83

Akrich, M. & B. Pasveer (2004) Embodiment and Disembodiment in Childbirth Narratives, *Body & Society*, vol. 10, 63–84

Appadurai, A. (1986) *The Social Life of Things: Commodities in Cultural Perspective*, Cambridge: Cambridge University Press

Armstrong, D. (1983) *Political Anatomy of the Body: Medical Knowledge in Britain in the Twentieth Century*, Cambridge: Cambridge University Press

Armstrong, D. (2002) *A New History of Identity: A Sociology of Medical Knowledge*, Basingstoke: Palgrave

Arney, W. & B. Bergen (1984) *Medicine and the Management of the Living: Taming the Last Great Beast*, Chicago, IL: University of Chicago Press

Ashmore, M., M. Mulkay & T. Pinch (1989) *Health and Efficiency: A Sociology of Health Economics*, Milton Keynes: Open University Press

Ashton, J. (1994) *The Epidemiological Imagination*, Milton Keynes: Open University Press

Bardbot, J. (2002) *Les Malades en mouvements: La médecine et la science à l'épreuve du sida*, Paris: Balland

Barnes, C., M. Oliver & L. Barton eds (2002) *Disability Studies Today*, Cambridge: Polity Press

Barry, A. (2001) *Political Machines: Governing a Technological Society*, London: Athlone

Becker, H. (1953) Becoming a Marihuana User, *American Journal of Sociology*, 59, 235–242

Berg, M. (1997) *Rationalizing Medicine: Decision Support Techniques and Medical Practices*, Cambridge, MA: MIT Press

Berg, M. & A. Mol eds (1998) *Differences in Medicine: Unraveling Practices, Techniques and Bodies*, Durham, NC: Duke University Press

Bingham, N. (2006) Bees, Butterflies, and Bacteria: Biotechnology and the Politics of Nonhuman Friendship, *Environment and Planning A* 38 (3), 483–498

Bliss, M. (1982) *The Discovery of Insulin*, Chicago, IL: University of Chicago Press

Böhme, G., W. v.d. Daele, R. Hohlfield, W. Krohn & W. Schäfer (1978) *Starn-*

berger Studien I: Die gesellschaftliche Orientierung des wissenschaftlichen Fortschritts, Frankfurt: Edition Suhrkamp

Boltanski, L. (1990) *L'Amour et la justice comme compétences*, Paris: Métalié

Bosk, C. (1979) *Forgive and Remember: Managing Medical Failure*, Chicago, IL: University of Chicago Press

Braak, E. ter (2000) *Insulin Induced Hypoglycemia and Glucose Counterregulations: Clinical and Experimental Studies*, Thesis: Utrecht University

Brah, A. & A. Coombes eds (2000) *Hybridity and Its Discontents: Politics, Science, Culture*, London: Routledge

Brown, N. & M. Michael (2003) Sociology of Expectations: Retrospecting Prospects and Prospecting Retrospects, *Technology Analysis and Strategic Management*, vol. 15 (1), 3–8

Burry, M. (2001) Illness Narratives: Fact or Fiction?, *Sociology of Health and Illness*, vol. 23, pp. 263–285

Callahan, D. & A. Wasunna eds (2006) *Medicine and the Market: Equity V. Choice*, Baltimore, MD: Johns Hopkins University Press

Callon, M. ed. (1998) *The Laws of the Market*, London: Blackwell

Callon, M. & V. Rabeharisoa (2004) Gino's Lesson on Humanity: Genetics, Mutual Entanglements and the Sociologist's Role, *Economy and Society*, vol. 33 (1), 1–27

Canguilhem, G. (1991) *The Normal and the Pathological*, New York: Zone Books

Canguilhem, G. (1994) *A Vital Rationalist*, New York: Zone Books

Chakrabarty, D. (2000) *Provincializing Europe: Postcolonial Thought and Historical Difference*, Princeton, NJ: Princeton University Press

Classen, C. (1993) *Worlds of Sense: Exploring the Senses in History and across Cultures*, London: Routledge

Cohn, S. (1997) Being Told What to Eat: Conversations in a Diabetes Day Centre, in P. Caplan ed., *Food, Health and Identity*, London: Routledge, pp. 193–212

Costera Meijer, I. (1991) Which Difference Makes the Difference? On the Conceptualization of Sexual Difference, in J. Hermsen & A. van Lenning eds, *Sharing the Difference: Feminist Debates in Holland*, London: Routledge, pp. 32–45

Coward, R. (1996) *Female Desire: Women's Sexuality Today*, London: HarperCollins

De Swaan, A. (1988) *In Care of the State: Health Care, Education and Welfare in Europe and America*, Cambridge: Polity Press

Dehue, T. (2005) History of the Control Group, in B. Everrit & D. Howel eds, *Encyclopedia of the Human Sciences*, vol. 2, 829–836

Despret, V. (2004) The Body We Care for: Figures of Anthropo-zoo-genesis, in *Body and Society*, vol. 10 (2–3), 111–134

Diedrich, L. (2005) A Bioethics of Failure: Anti-heroic Cancer Narratives, in M. Shildrick & R. Mykitiuk eds, *Ethics of the Body: Postconventional Challenges*, Cambridge, MA: MIT Press

Dodier, N. (1993) *L'expertise médical*, Paris: Métaillié

Dodier, N. (1998) Clinical Practice and Procedures in Occupational Medicine: A Study of the Framing of Individuals, in M. Berg & A. Mol eds, *Differences in Medicine: Unraveling Practices, Techniques and Bodies*, Durham, NC: Duke University Press, pp. 53–85

Dodier, N. (2003) *Leçons politiques de l'épidemie de sida*, Paris: Éditions de l'École des Hautes Études en Sciences Sociales

Duden, B. (2002) *Die Gene im Kopf – der Fötus im Bauch*, Hanover: Offizin Verlag

Duster, T. (2003) *Backdoor to Eugenics*, New York: Routledge

Elias, N. (2000) *The Civilizing Process*, Oxford: Blackwell

Epstein, S. (1996) *Impure Science : Aids, Activism and the Politics of Knowledge*, Berkeley: University of California Press

Farmer, P. (2004) *Pathologies of Power: Health, Human Rights and the New War on the Poor*, Berkeley: University of California Press

Foucault, M. (1967) *Madness and Civilisation*, London: Tavistock

Foucault, M. (1974) *The Order of Things: An Archeology of the Human Sciences*, London: Tavistock

Foucault, M. (1976) *The Birth of the Clinic*, trans. A. Smith, London: Tavistock

Foucault, M. (1986) Of Other Spaces, *Diactrics*, vol. 6 (1), 22–27

Foucault, M. (1990) *Care of the Self: The History of Sexuality 3*, trans. R. Hurley, London: Penguin

Foucault, M. (1991) *Discipline and Punish*, trans. A. Sheridan, London: Penguin

Frank, A. (1991) *At the Will of the Body*, Boston, MA: Houghton Mifflin Company

Frank, A. (1995) *The Wounded Storyteller: Body, Illness and Ethics*, Chicago, IL: University of Chicago Press

Frank, A. (2004) *The Renewal of Generosity: Illness, Medicine and How to Live*, Chicago, IL: The University of Chicago Press

Frankenberg, R. (1993) Risk: Anthropological and Epidemiological Narratives of Prevention, in S. Lindenbaum & M. Lock eds, *Knowledge, Power and Practice*, Berkeley: University of California Press, pp. 219–244

Freidson, E. (2001) *Professionalism: The Third Logic*, London: Cambridge Polity Press

Freudtner, C. (2003) *Bittersweet: Diabetes, Insulin and the Transformation of Illness*, University of North Carolina Press

Gatens, M. (1996) *Imaginary Bodies: Ethics, Power and Corporeality*, London: Routledge

Gigerenzer, G. *et al.* (1989) *The Empire of Chance: How Probability Changed Science and Everyday Life*, Cambridge: Cambridge University Press

Golledge, R. (1997) On Reassembling One's Life: Overcoming Disability in the Academic Environment, *Environment and Planning D: Society and Space*, 15, 391–409

Gomart, E. & A. Hennion (1999) A Sociology of Attachment: Music Amateurs, Drug Users, in J. Law & J. Hassard eds, *Actor Network Theory and After*, Oxford: Blackwell, pp. 220–247

Goodman, A., D. Heath & M. Lindee (2003) *Genetic Nature/Culture*, Berkeley: University of California Press

Goody, J. (1986) *The Logic of Writing and the Organization of Society*, Cambridge: Cambridge University Press

Greenhalgh, T. & B. Hurwitz (1998) *Narrative-Based Medicine*, London: BMJ Books

Hacking, I. (1990) *The Taming of Chance*, Cambridge: Cambridge University Press

Haeften T. van (1995) Acute complicaties – hypoglykemische ontregeling, in E. van Ballegooie & R. Heine eds, *Diabetes Mellitus*, Ultrecht: Wetenschappelijke Uitgeverij Bunge, pp. 142–150

Hahn, R. (1985) A World of Internal Medicine: Portrait of an Internist, in R. Hahn & A. Gaines eds, *Physicians of Western Medicine: Anthropological Approaches to Theory and Practice*, Dordrecht: Reidel Publishing Group, pp. 51–111

Hamington, M. & D. Miller eds (2006) *Socializing Care*, Oxford: Rowman & Littlefield

Haraway, D. (1997) *Modest Witness*, London: Routledge

Haraway, D. (2003) *The Companion Species Manifesto: Dogs, People and Significant Otherness*, Chicago, IL: Chicago University Press

Harbers, H., A. Mol & A. Stollmeijer (2002) Food Matters. Arguments for an Ethnography of Daily Care, *Theory, Culture and Society*, vol. 19 (5/6), 207–226

Healy, D. (2004) *The Creation of Psychofarmacology*, Cambridge, MA: Harvard University Press

Hennion, A. (2001) Music Lovers: Taste as Performance, *Theory, Culture and Society*, Vol. 18 (5), 1–22

Herzlich, C. & J. Pierret (1984) *Malades d'hier, malades d'aujourdhui*, Paris: Payot

Hinchliffe, S. (2008) Reconstituting Nature Conservation: Towards a Careful Political Ecology, *Geoforum*, vol. 39 (1), 88–97

Hirschauer, S. (1994) The Manufacture of Bodies in Surgery, *Social Studies of Science*, vol. 21, 279–319

Hirschauer, S. (2005) On Doing Being a Stranger: The Practical Constitution of Civil Inattention, *Journal for the Theory of Social Behaviour*, 35 (1), 41–67

Hirschauer, H. & A. Mol (1995) Shifting Sexes, Moving Stories: Constructivist/Feminist Dialogues, *Science, Technology and Human Values*, vol. 20, 368–385

Hoesset, E. (2003) *L'intelligence de la pitié*, Paris: Les Éditions du Cerf

Hoeyer, K. (2006) The Power of Ethics: A Case Study from Sweden on the Social Life of Moral Concerns in Policy Processes, *Sociology of Health and Illness*, vol. 28, 785–801

Howarth, D., A. Norval & Y. Stavrakakis eds (2000) *Discourse Theory and Political Analysis*, Manchester: Manchester University Press

Howell, S. ed. (1997) *The Ethnography of Moralities*, London: Routledge

Ingstad, B. & V. Christie (2001) Encounters with Illness: The Perspective of the Sick Doctor, *Anthropology and Medicine*, vol. 8, 201–210

James, S. (1999) *Passion and Action: The Emotions in Seventeenth Century Philosophy*, Oxford: Oxford University Press

Julien, F. (2001) *Detour and Access: Strategies of Meaning in China and Greece*, New York: Zone Books

Kleinman, A. (1980) *Patients and Healers in the Context of Culture*, Berkeley: University of California Press

Kleinman, A., V. Das & M. Lock eds (1997) *Social Suffering*, Berkeley: University of California Press

Kondo, D. (1990) *Crafting Selves: Power, Gender, and Discourses of Identity in a Japanese Workplace*, Chicago, IL: University of Chicago Press

Kurlyama, S. (1999) *The Expressiveness of the Body: And the Divergence of Greek and Chinese Medicine*, New York: Zone Books

Laet, M. de & A. Mol (2000) The Zimbabwe Bush Pump: Mechanics of a Fluid Technology, *Social Studies of Science*, vol. 30, pp. 225–263

Lakoff, A. (2006) *Pharmaceutical Reason: Knowledge and Value in Global Psychiatry*, Cambridge: Cambridge University Press

Lakoff, G. & M. Johnson (1981) *Metaphors We Live By*, Chicago, IL: University of Chicago Press

Lakoff, G. & M. Johnson (1999) *Philosophy of in the Flesh: The Embodied Mind and Its Challenge to Western Thought*, New York: Basic Books

Latour, B. (1988) *The Pasteurization of France*, Cambridge, MA: Harvard University Press

Latour, B. (1996) *Aramis or the Love of Technology*, Cambridge, MA: Harvard University Press

Latour, B. (2002) Morality and Technology: The End of the Means, *Theory, Culture & Society*, vol. 19 (5/6), 247–260

Latour, B. (2004) Why Has Critique Run out of Steam? From Matters of Fact to Matters of Concern, *Critical Inquiry*, vol. 30, 225–248

Latour, B. & P. Weibel eds (2005) *Making Things Public*, Cambridge, MA: MIT Press

Latour, B. & S. Woolgar (1979) *Laboratory Life: The Social Construction of Scientific Facts*, London: Sage Publications

LaVeist, T. ed. (2002) *Race, Ethnicity, and Health: A Public Health Reader*, Hoboker, NJ: Jossey-Bass

Law, J. (1994) *Organizing Modernity*, Oxford: Blackwell

Law, J. (2002) *Aircraft Stories: Decentering the Object in Technoscience*, Durham, NC: Duke University Press

Law, J. (2004) *After Method: Mess In Social Science Research*, London: Routledge

Law, J. & A. Mol (2002) Local Entanglements or Utopian Moves: An Inquiry into Train Accidents, in M. Parker ed., *Utopia and Organization*, Oxford: Blackwell *Sociological Review*, pp. 82–105

Lawrence, C. & S. Shapin eds (1998) *Science Incarnate: Historical Embodiments of Natural Knowledge*, Chicago, IL: University of Chicago Press

Lettinga, L. & A. Mol (1999) Clinical Specificity and the Non-generalities of Science: On Innovation Strategies for Neurological Physical Therapy, *Theoretical Medicine and Bioethics*, 1999, 517–535

Lifton, R. (1988) *The Nazi Doctors: Medical Killing and the Psychology of Genocide*, New York: Basic Books

Lin, W.-Y. (2005) *Bodies in Action: Multivalent Agency in Haemodialysis Practices*, Lancaster, PhD thesis

Lock, M. (2002) *Twice Dead: Organ Transplants and the Reinvention of Death*, Berkeley: University of California Press

Lock, M., A. Young & A. Cambriosio eds (2000) *Living and Working with The New Medical Technologies: Intersections of Inquiry*, Cambridge: Cambridge University Press

Lury, C. (1996) *Consumer Culture*, London: Routledge

Marks, H. (1997) *The Progress of Experiment: Science and Therapeutic Reform in the United States, 1900–1990*, Cambridge: Cambridge University Press

Martin, E. (2006) Pharmaceutical Virtue, *Medicine, Culture and Society*, vol. 30 (2), 157–174

Mauss, M. (1990) *The Gift*, trans. W. Halls, London: Routledge

M'charek, A. (2005) *The Human Genome Diversity Project: An Ethnography of Scientific Practice*, Cambridge: Cambridge University Press

Meneley, A. & D. Young eds (2005) *Auto-ethnographies: The Anthropology of Academic Practices*, Ontario: Broadview Press

Michael, M. (2006) *Technoscience and Everyday Life*, Milton Keynes: Open University Press

Mintz, S. (1985) *Sweetness and Power: The Place of Sugar in Modern History*, London: Penguin

Mintz, S. (1996) *Tasting Food, Tasting Freedom: Excursions into Eating, Culture and the Past*, Boston, MA: Beacon Press

Mol, A. (1991) Wombs, Pigmentation and Pyramids. Should Anti-racists and Feminists Try to Confine Biology to Its Proper Place?, in A. van Lenning & J. Hermsen eds, *Sharing the Difference: Feminist Debates in Holland*, London: Routledge, pp. 149–163

Mol, A. (1998) Lived Reality and the Multiplicity of Norms: A Critical Tribute to George Canguilhem, *Economy and Society*, vol. 27, 274–284

Mol, A. (1999) Ontological Politics: A Word and Some Questions, in J. Law and J. Hassard eds, *Actor Network Theory and After*, Oxford: Blackwell, pp. 74–89

Mol, A. (2002a) *The Body Multiple: Ontology in Medical Practice*, Durham, NC: Duke University Press

Mol, A. (2002b) Cutting Surgeons, Walking Patients: Some Complexities Involved in Comparing, in J. Law and A. Mol eds, *Complexities*, Durham, NC: Duke University Press, pp. 218–257

Mol, A. & M. Berg (1994) Principles and Practices of Medicine: The Co-existence of Various Anemias, *Culture, Medicine and Psychiatry*, vol. 18, 247–265

Mol, A. & B. Elsman (1996) Detecting Disease and Designing Treatment: Duplex and the Diagnosis of Diseased Leg Vessels, *Sociology of Health and Illness*, vol. 18 (5), 609–631

Mol, A. & J. Law (1994) Regions, Networks and Fluids: Anemia and Social Topology, *Social Studies of Science*, 24, 641–671

Mol, A. & J. Law (2004) Embodied Action, Enacted Bodies: The Example of Hypoglycaemia, *Body & Society*, vol. 10 (2–3), 43–62

Moreira, T. (2004) Self, Agency and the Surgical Collective, *Sociology of Health & Illness*, vol. 26 (1), 32–49

Moreira, T. (2006) Heterogeneity and Coordination of Blood Pressure in Neurosurgery, *Social Studies of Science*, vol. 36 (1), 69–97

Moreira, T. & P. Palladino (2005) Between Truth and Hope on Parkinson's Disease, Neurotransplantation and the Production of the Self, *History of the Human Sciences*, vol. 18 (3), 55–82

Morse, J., I. Bottoff, W. Neander & S. Sorberg (1992) Comparative Analysis of Conceptualizations and Theories of Caring, in J. Morse ed., *Qualitative Health Research*, Newbury Park, CA: Sage, pp. 69–89

Moser, I. (2006) Sociotechnical Practices and Differences: On the Interferences between Disability, Gender and Class, *Science, Technology and Human Values*, vol. 31 (5), 1–28

Murphy, R. (1990) *The Body Silent*, New York: W.W. Norton

Nabhan, P. (2006) *Why Some Like It Hot: Food, Genes and Cultural Diversity*, Washington, DC: Island Press

Nestle, M. (2002) *Food Politics: How the Food Industry Influences Nutrition and Health*, Berkeley: University of California Press

Nussbaum, M & A. Sen eds (1993) *The Quality of Life*, Oxford: Clarendon Press

Nye, A. (1990) *Words of Power: A Feminist Reading of the History of Logic*, London: Routledge

Okely, J. & H. Callaway (1992) *Anthropology and Autobiography*, London: Routledge

Oudshoorn, N. & T. Pinch eds (2005) *How Users Matter: The Co-Construction of Users and Technology*, Cambridge, MA: MIT Press

Parsons, T. (1951) *The Social System*, New York: Free Press

Pasveer, B. (1992) *Shadows of Knowledge: Making a Representing Practice in Medicine: X-ray Pictures and Pulmonary Tuberculosis, 1895–1930*, Amsterdam: PhD thesis

Petryna, A. (2002) *Life Exposed: Biological Citizens after Chernobyl*, Princeton, NJ: Princeton University Press

Pickstone, J. (2000) *Ways of Knowing: A New History of Science, Technology and Medicine*, Manchester: Manchester University Press

Pignarre, P. (1997) *Quest-ce qu'un médicament? Un object étrange, entre science, marché et société*, Paris: Éditions le Découverte

Pols, J. (2003) Enforcing Patient Rights of Improving Care? The Interference of Two Modes of Doing Good in Mental Health Care, *Sociology of Health and Illness*, vol. 25 (4), 320–347

Pols, J. (2005) Enacting Appreciations: Beyond the Patient Perspective, *Health Care Analysis*, vol. 13, 203–221

Pols, J. (2006a) Accounting and Washing, *Science, Technology & Human Values*, vol. 31 (4), 409–430

Pols, J. (2006b) Washing the Citizen: Washing, Cleanliness and Citizenship in Mental Health Care, *Culture, Medicine and Psychiatry*, vol. 30, 77–104

Prior, L. (1989) *The Social Organization of Death: Medical Discourse and Social Practices in Belfast*, Houndsmills: Macmillan

Rabeharisoa, V. & M. Callon (1999) *Le Pouvoir des malades*, Presse de l'École de Mînes

Rabinow, P. & N. Rose (2006) Biopower Today, *BioSocieties*, vol. 1, 195–217

Reiser, S. (1978) *Medicine and the Reign of Technology*, Cambridge: Cambridge University Press

Reiser, S. & M. Anbar eds (1984) *The Machine at the Bedside: Strategies of Using Technology in Patient Care*, Cambridge: Cambridge University Press

Rip, A., T. Misa & J. Schot eds (1995) *Managing Technology in Society: The Approach of Constructive Technology Assessment*, London: Thomson Learning

Robinson, F. (1998) *Globalising Care: Feminist Theory, Ethics and International Relations*, Boulder, CO: Westview Press

Rock, M. (2003) Sweet Blood and Social Suffering: Rethinking Cause–Effect Relationships in Diabetes, Distress, and Duress, *Medical Anthropology*, vol. 22 (2), 131–174

Rock, M. (2005) Figuring Out Type 2 Diabetes through Genetic Research: Reckoning Kinship and the Origins of Sickness, *Anthropology & Medicine*, vol. 12 (2), 115–127

Roney, L. (2000) *Sweet Invisible Body: Reflections on a Life with Diabetes*, New York: Owl Books

Sacks, O. (1984) A Leg to Stand on, London: Picador Books

Saïd, E. (1991) *Orientalism: Western Conceptions of the Orient*, London: Penguin

Santoro, E. (2004) *Autonomy, Freedom and Rights: A Critique of Liberal Subjectivity*, Dordrecht: Kluwer

Schwartz, B. (2004) *The Paradox of Choice: Why More Is Less*, London: HarperCollins

Scott, J. (1999) *Gender and the Politics of History*, New York: Columbia University Press

Serres, M. (1997) *The Troubadour of Knowledge*, trans. S. Glaser & W. Paulson, Ann Arbor: University of Michigan Press

Serres, M. (2007) *Parasite*, Minneapolis: University of Minnesota Press

Shakespeare, T. (2006) *Disability Rights and Wrongs*, London: Routledge

Shapin, S. (2000) Descartes the Doctor: Rationalism and its Therapies, *British Journal for the History of Science*, 33, 131–154

Shaw, R. (2000) Tok Af, Lef Af: A Political Economy of Temne Techniques of Secrecy and Self, in I. Karp & D.A. Masolo eds, *African Philosophy as Cultural Inquiry*, Bloomington: Indiana University Press, pp. 25–49

Smith, B. (1981) Black Lung: The Social Production of a Disease, *International Journal of Health Services*, 11, 343–359

Solnit, R. (2006) *Wanderlust: A History of Walking*, London: Verso

Ssorin-Chaikov (2006) On Heterochrony: Birthday Gifts to Stalin, 1949, *Journal of the Royal Anthropological Institute*, vol. 12, 355–375

Stacey, J. (1997) *Teratologies: A Cultural Study of Cancer*, London: Routledge

Stein, H. (1990) *American Medicine as Culture*. Boulder, CO: Westview Press

Stengers, I. (1998) *Power and Invention: Situating Science*, Minneapolis: University of Minnesota Press

Strathern, M. (1988) *The Gender of the Gift*, Berkeley: University of California Press

Strathern, M. (1992) *After Nature: English Kinship in the Late Twentieth Century*, Cambridge: Cambridge University Press

Strauss, A., S. Fagerhaugh, B. Suczek and C. Wiener (1985) *Social Organization of Medical Work*, Chicago, IL: University of Chicago Press

Struhkamp, R. (2004) Goals in Their Setting: A Normative Analysis of Goal Setting in Physical Rehabilitation, *Health Care Analysis*, vol. 12, 131–155

Struhkamp, R. (2005a) Patient Autonomy: A View from the Kitchen, *Medicine, Health Care and Philosophy*, vol. 8, 105–114

Struhkamp, R. (2005b) Wordless Pain: Dealing with Suffering in Physical Rehabilitation, *Cultural Studies*, vol. 19, pp. 701–718

Sunder Rajan, K. (2006) *Biocapital: The Constitution of Postgenomic Life*, Durham, NC: Duke University Press

Svare, H. (2005) *Body and Practice in Kant*, Dordrecht: Kluwer Academic Publishers

Taylor, J. (2005) Surfacing the Body Interior, *Annual Review of Anthropology*, 34, 741–756

Teil, G. (2004) *De la coupe au lèvres: Practiques de la perception et mise en marché de vins de qualité*, Paris: Octares

Thévenot, L. (2002) Which Road to Follow? The Moral Complexity of an Equipped Humanity, in J. Law & A. Mol eds, *Complexities: Social Studies of Knowledge Practice*, Durham, NC: Duke University Press, pp. 35–87

Thévenot, L. (2006) *L'action au pluriel: Sociologie des régimes dengagement*, Paris: Éditions de la Découverte

Thomas, N. (1991) *Entangled Objects: Exchange, Material Culture and Colonialism in the Pacific*, Cambridge, MA: Harvard University Press

Thompson, C. (2005) *Making Parents: The Ontological Choreography of Reproductive Technologies*, Cambridge, MA: MIT Press

Toulmin, S. (1998) How Medicine Saved the Life of Ethics, in J. DeMarco & R. Fox eds, *New Directions in Ethics: The Challenge of Applied Ethics*, London: Routledge and Kegan Paul, pp. 265–281

Tronto, J. (1993) *Moral Boundaries: A Political Argument for an Ethic of Care*, New York/London: Routledge

Tudor Hart, J. (2006) *The Political Economy of Health Care: A Clinical Perspective*, Bristol: Policy Press

Vallega-Neu, D. (2005) *The Bodily Dimension in Thinking*, New York: State of New York University Press

Varela, F. (2001) Intimate Distances: Fragments for a Phenomenology of Organ Transplantation, *Journal of Consciousness Studies*, vol. 8, 5–7

Verran, H. (2001) *Science and an African Logic*, Chicago, IL: University of Chicago Press

Vries, G. de & K. Horstman, eds (2007) *Genetics from Laboratory to Society*, Basingstoke: Palgrave Macmillan

Walzer, M. (1983) *Spheres of Justice: A Defence of Pluralism and Equality*, Oxford: Blackwell

Watson, J. & M. Caldwell eds (2005) *The Cultural Politics of Food and Eating*, Oxford: Blackwell

Weisz, G. ed. (1990) *Social Science Perspectives on Medical Ethics*, Dordrecht: Kluwer Academic Publishers

Willems, D. (1998) Inhaling Drugs and Making Worlds: The Proliferation of Lungs and Asthmas, in M. Berg & A. Mol eds, *Differences in Medicine: Unraveling Practices, Techniques and Bodies*, Durham, NC: Duke University Press

Willems, D. (2002) Managing One's Body Using Self-management Techniques: Practicing Autonomy, *Theoretical Medicine and Bioethics*, vol. 31 (1), 23–38

Winance, M. (2006) Trying Out the Wheelchair: The Mutual Shaping of People and Devices through Adjustment, *Science, Technology & Human Values*, vol. 31 (1), 52–72

Woolgar, S. (1991) Configuring the User: The Case of Usability Trials, in J. Law ed., *A Sociology of Monsters*, London: Routledge, pp. 57–102

Wright, P. & A. Treacher eds (1982) *The Problem of Medical Knowledge: Examining the Social Construction of Medicine*, Edinburgh: Edinburgh University Press

Xperiment! (2005) What Is a Body/a Person? Topography of the Possible, in B. Latour & P. Weibel eds, *Making Things Public*, Cambridge, MA: MIT Press, pp. 906–909

Index

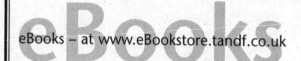

Printed in the United States
by Baker & Taylor Publisher Services